MW00877875

TRANSCENDING MS

MARGIE HUNTER

ISBN: 978-1-4834-6021-5 (sc)
ISBN: 978-1-4834-6022-2 (e)

Library of Congress Control Number: 2016917302

Images by Kristin Hunter

Lulu Publishing Services rev. date: 12/12/2016

Preface

If you are reading this it is probably because you have MS or someone you care about does. I am so sorry you have to go through this, but there is hope. I was diagnosed in 1999. I can now say I *had* MS. Today I am healthy and strong. I have written this book with the intention to help anyone with MS also become healthy and strong. There are two parts in this book: you get to know me in Part One, and in Part Two you will get to know you. It is a simple and straightforward guide to healing. Along with the book, you will have access to my website and e-mail to help with the process. Any unanswered questions along the way will ultimately be answered. Video and audio clips will be available as guides at transcendingms.com. The whole process is designed to support you on your way to regaining balance and health in your life.

Thank you for joining me in my effort to help you. We can do this together.

With love,
Margie Hunter

Introduction

I'm not a doctor, nor an expert. I am just a woman who one day was told she had multiple sclerosis. What came after was very complicated and complex, but I managed to work my way through it. I don't claim to be special. I am just like you. What happened to me along the way to health is nothing short of incredible. I believe I got sick so I could help you. So here we are. Together we can and will overcome and transcend.

On the surface this story is about my life with multiple sclerosis. Yes it's that. But, more importantly it is the story followed by a guide to live with and without MS, because MS has lost its impact on my life. The truth of the matter is that all I'm about to tell you could apply to any and all diseases in their varying forms. But I can only speak of my experience, and my experience is with MS.

My acceptance, and then subsequent release, of the *dis-ease* has led to many paths in my life I would have never followed otherwise. As strange as it may sound, it's been a blessing to me. I've learned the importance of embracing and living every moment of my life. I am human and sometimes almost slip into old habits—the same habits that I believe brought on my illness—but the effort to live in the *now* is ever important. There was a time, when I was diagnosed and very sick, when it was all very hard. I know about waking up in the morning and being angry and scared about my future. I know about the feeling of helplessness and sadness. I know about wanting to give up and fall into depression. But, I have also been blessed with people and signs in my life that have guided me to recognize a different and healing path. I've tried not to let things pass me by without taking a second look at them. I've found that circumstances have been placed in my path to help me. It has been up to me to use them and help myself. Until we make the decision to help ourselves and leave the disease behind, it won't leave us. Make a deliberate and conscious effort to affirm and reaffirm your decision to not have MS be a part of you anymore. I know you may be thinking, "This nut-job doesn't know what she's talking about!" Well, with all my heart and soul, I can tell you that I have been there and have worked my way to balance and health—and I want to help you to do the same. We are put on this earth to help each other, and if I can help you through this book, my getting sick will have been worth it. Let me, and this book, be among the signs placed in your path to help you.

CHAPTER 1

The Fall of the People Pleaser

I'm not sure where to start. Until now, I haven't really sat down to delve into the specifics of the beginning of my journey with MS. Or to recall and look into all the emotions and just how sick and scared I was. I have focused on getting better and wanting to help others do so as well. But in order to help you, I was convinced by my daughter that I needed to tell you my story. My story with all its ups and downs and in-betweens. So, this is it. This is the story of a woman, that woman being me, who got very sick in the prime of her life. By all accounts I had everything any woman could ever want and more. Little did I know, the price I was paying for it.

It was 1998 and I was thirty-eight years-old. I had three children. My oldest was a beautiful, spunky 13 year-old girl. A teenager with all the headaches that come with a typical teenager. My second beautiful, brilliant child was a 12 year-old girl on her way to being a teenager and giving me a run for my money. My very beautiful, gentle son was two and giving me so much joy I could hardly believe it. They were all the joy of my life. I was married to my other joy. My life was everything I wanted. I lived exactly where I wanted to live. My children went to the schools where I wanted them to go. I set up my life so I could structure my work schedule around my children's schedule. We owned our own business so I was very lucky to be able to do that. I was well aware of how lucky I was, and as a result, I thought I owed it to my family and all those around me to do as much as I could to make their lives better. I would get up in the morning and between my husband and I, we would get the kids fed, ready for school and I would put all three in the car and take the two oldest to school. My son and I would go to my office. I would work and he would play. Some days I would go to his co-op preschool with him, swim lessons and then of course many play dates. In the afternoons we would pick up his sisters and that's when our days would really begin. There were many after-school activities to drive them to and homework to be done, and endless philanthropic activities in a mother-daughter organization. We were all very, very busy.

I was involved in my children's lives from the moment they were born in what I thought was an exceptional way. I taught them how to swim in *Mommy and Me* classes. I sat through days, months and years of gymnastics classes, swim team, karate, softball and basketball and so many others. I was "room mother," Girl Scout leader and I would teach Spanish to them in their preschool and throughout their primary school classes. To be honest, that is just a glimpse of all the organized volunteering I did with and without them. There were not many moments of rest. But I loved being with my kids and had an ideal life.

I played tennis year-round. In the summer I windsurfed. In the winter we spent a lot of time skiing. I loved to be outdoors any chance I got. I was very busy keeping myself in shape and loving every minute of it. It was my escape from all the responsibilities that became at times overwhelming.

Beginning in about 1993 my father's health started declining. He spent a lot of time in and out of the hospital. He seemed to be on the verge of dying over and over. Then suddenly making unexpected miraculous recoveries. As a result I spent many, many nights at the hospital with him over the course of five years. After finishing all the activities with the kids, my husband would take over for me and I would sit in the hospital for a few hours a night. It was a hard and very lonely time. I have no siblings and no other family to share these incredibly painful and stressful times as they happened. I had to be strong and not let on how difficult all of this was for me. Only my husband knew what this was doing to me. By 1998, my father was spending more time in, rather than out of the hospital.

So as you can see, I was an over achiever. I wanted to be a perfect mother, perfect wife, perfect daughter, perfect businesswoman, perfect all-around in anything and everything I did. Unfortunately the impossibility of this was escaping me at that time. I was a people pleaser and didn't know it. I always thought of myself as independent, someone who never cared what others thought, but I had fallen in the trap of thinking of myself as indispensable and did not know how to say "no." Who better for any job than me? Even for the things I didn't want to do, there was a *yes* and never a *no*. I was taking on more and more regardless of whether I had the space for it. Needless to say, this was a formula for disaster.

I don't know how that happened. Thinking back on the way things were when I was first married may give a clue. The plan was that my husband, Mark, and I would go to London 9 months after getting married. I had just finished college and was going to work for the BBC and Mark was going to attend London School of Economics for his graduate work. A month after we were married, we found out I was pregnant. Our plans had to change. How was I going to tell Dad?

I was an only child of parents who divorced by the time I was five years-old. I lived with my mother during the school year and spent summers with my father. His expectations of me as a child were always very high. His expectations of me after my teenage years were very low. Although I was a bright girl, I did not spend a lot of time studying in high school. I was more interested in socializing and dancing than hitting the books. By that point, my father was convinced I wouldn't amount to much. I had been living with my mother and didn't really know him well, until I moved close to him to go to college. I had to prove myself over and over to him throughout my college career. Once my father realized I actually could excel and succeed in anything I put my mind to, his standards for me rose and the pressure was on. He wanted me to be a career woman and to achieve quite a bit in my life before having children. The pregnancy was, of course, not expected and he flipped his lid when I told him. For months before having the baby he would visit and give me the divorce statistics for California, which were alarmingly high. In his mind, I was on my way to becoming a single mother.

We moved for a job opportunity for Mark. I, on the other, hand had no job and it was not likely that I could get a job very easily as pregnant as I was. So, Dad helped me start my own translation business. I had worked for a Language School while I was in college, and I was fluent in English and Spanish with experience teaching and translating. "This will be a piece of cake for me," I thought. The truth of the matter is that I had no idea how I was going to manage it.

I had brochures designed and printed. Then sent out ten brochures to different advertising agencies and, lo and behold, I got lucky and landed an incredible contract translating and dubbing T.V. commercials for a large company. At this point I was about five months pregnant, but looked like I was going to deliver any minute. My clients would pray during that time that I would be able to get things to them without the baby coming. I managed to figure it out. I found a studio for the voice-overs, another one to lay the soundtrack on videos, and I found talent to do the voices. After Mark got home from work I would go to the studio for a few hours to record and edit voices. The next day the sound would go onto the video. I had no professional production experience, but I made it work. The client loved the first project and this meant steady work every month from the same agency for their commercials. It was important for me to succeed in this, not only to help financially, but also to prove to my father that I could be the Super Woman he expected me to be. This began translating into every part of my life. In every area in my life, I felt the pressure to go above and beyond; I needed to be *more* than I felt I was. From how I raised my children, to how I ran my business, became a challenge at all times and doubting myself and striving for perfection at all times. For many years no matter what I did it was never good enough. So I kept filling my plate hoping someday that recognition would come. It did come, but by then my plate was so full it was cracking. This pace continued for 13 years.

So I come back to an afternoon in 1998. I had been busily going about my day with the kids, work, and everything else. Somehow I got a rare chance to take a much-needed nap. I slipped upstairs to my room, lay down and fell asleep. A little while later I woke up from a very deep sleep. I opened my eyes and something felt odd. I couldn't feel my right eye. I couldn't feel the right side of my lip. It didn't stop there. I couldn't feel the right side of my nose, my cheek, my forehead, my ear or my scalp on that side. The right side of my head was completely numb. I sat up in bed and waited to see if it would pass. Maybe I had slept in a weird position and that was why. I stood up to see if that would make a difference. I went to the mirror to see if my face showed signs of anything wrong. I looked for a droopy eye or a droopy lip. Nope—I looked perfectly normal, which was even stranger. I stood at the window looking out, waiting for it to pass, but it didn't. I tried to think if maybe there was something I had done that could be causing this to happen. I had been to the dentist a couple of weeks before, could that be it? I got on the phone and called my dentist's office and told them what was happening to me, but they didn't think the dental work had anything to do with it. What to do next? I didn't want to alarm anyone. I kept thinking it would go away, but it didn't. A little bit of panic was starting to run through me. What could possibly be wrong?

Nothing else was happening to me, so I was able to stay calm, but I still wanted to get to the bottom of what was happening. Looking back now, had I been more aware, I would have recognized other signs that had been happening to me—little things that made me feel like something was wrong. So I called my doctor and set up a visit.

Aside from being my doctor, he is also a friend, so I was happy to be sitting there. After relaying my symptoms, and at that time the only symptom was the numbness in my face and head, he asked many questions. Finally, because that was really the only concrete symptom I had, my doctor came to the conclusion I had a virus settle on a cluster of nerves above the right ear, which is the command center for feeling on that side of the face and head. He walked out of the room and came back with a book showing exactly where they were. He said the feeling would come back as soon as the virus went away. I was so relieved and so happy. Thank goodness!

As days passed the numbness didn't go away. Everyone I talked to about it had a story of someone they knew who had something like that happen to them, and they were fine. From my hair dresser to the gardener, everyone knew a case like mine. No one seemed the least bit alarmed by it. In fact, I was feeling fine other than that, so I was more at ease with what was happening to me, strange as it all was. I didn't tell the kids about it. It didn't seem necessary for them to know. Why alarm them if there was nothing wrong?

A few weeks later it was Thanksgiving week and we had a trip planned for our family. We packed up the car with a turkey and all the trimmings to prepare and headed for a ski vacation in Mammoth, California. We loved skiing and we all loved Mammoth. I was so much looking forward to it. Fresh powder, sunny skies, and my beautiful family. It didn't get better than that. We reached the condo and unpacked. It was our first snow trip of the year and the girls were very excited to start playing in the snow. I went out with them and we played and played. The boys followed us and were having a great time, throwing snowballs, making angels and slushing through the powder. The girls and I decided to run up a hill. We were all busy being silly. As we decided to head back the girls ran down to the bottom of the hill ahead of me. I was getting up from where I was in the snow to run behind them and I lost my balance and fell. *Whoa!* There's a moment in life where everything changes, and for me, this was it. It was a moment of complete helplessness and confusion. Out of left field came an imbalance like nothing I had ever felt.

I don't know exactly how long, but it took some time to regain my bearings and scoot my way down the hill on my backside. Standing up felt impossible. When I finally got to the bottom, I gave it everything I had and finally got to my feet. I was unsteady, light-headed, and a little dizzy. Maybe the virus had gone into my ear. Maybe the altitude was affecting me.

Needless to say, I spent the weekend indoors watching it snow outside. In fact, the girls got sick and my son didn't ski, so we all spent the days together playing games and watching television while Mark skied. I was slightly out of commission, so everyone participated in cooking Thanksgiving dinner. It was a very joyous occasion. I felt I was the luckiest woman in the world to be surrounded by these incredible beings I loved so much. I absolutely loved being a mom and a wife. A little virus couldn't put a damper on my favorite holiday. I had so much to be grateful for. As the weekend came to an end, we packed up and left for home. I was still light-headed, and tired, but I figured once at sea level I would feel better.

Once we got home from the mountains I headed straight for bed. I was tired and really not feeling very well. I still felt dizzy if I moved quickly, so everything I did had to be at a slow pace. The next morning I got up and immediately fell. I had extreme vertigo and couldn't walk. I felt nauseous and needed to vomit. I made my way to the bathroom and tried to control what was happening to me but couldn't. Somehow I let Mark know what was happening. He drove me to the doctor as everything was spinning around me.

Once in the parking lot, Mark had to help me walk to the doctor's office. I don't know how we managed. It seemed like an impossible distance for me. My doctor checked me out and didn't have too much to say. We needed to stop the vertigo that was making me so violently ill, so he prescribed some medications to keep me comfortable and ordered an MRI immediately. At this point my vision was becoming blurred and I couldn't focus on anything, but I thought it was because of the vertigo.

CHAPTER 2

Losing My Independence

Everything seemed so surreal to me. One minute I was running around getting along with my life and the next minute I was in a terrifying position for no apparent reason. This is when I realized how quickly life can change. Thank God I had Mark. I had been the rock for everyone in my life up to that point. It felt so good to know that I had a rock to lean on. I had always felt that I could handle anything, that I was invincible in many ways. So now I was completely helpless. Something I had never been before.

I had never had an MRI and suffered from claustrophobia. The idea of lying in an enclosed space for any length of time sounded like torture to me, but there was no other way. Many thoughts were running through my mind. I wondered if I had a brain tumor, or maybe I had some other horrible disease going on in my brain. My doctor prescribed something to help keep me calm during the time in the tube.

As much as I didn't want to, I went to the radiology center for the MRI. My memories of this are few, but the ones I have are very vivid. After spending some time in the waiting room with incredible fear and anxiety, they took me to a small room to change and put away all my belongings. I changed into a robe, walked into a room separated from all human contact and went in the MRI tube. I had never been sick so all of this seemed to be something out of a movie—but worse. It was happening to me.

I felt so alone lying there, and more afraid than I'd been in my life. It was all so strange. As I lay there trying not to cry, a voice would come on and ask me to be still. *Still?* I didn't know I had moved! Time passed very slowly in the tube as a loud banging and buzzing went on for what seemed like hours. Thoughts were running through my head: *Why is this happening? How am I going to explain this to my parents? How am I going to explain this to my kids?* I had too much to do; three kids, a husband, an extremely ill father, and a whole host of responsibilities I had committed to. How was I in this position when just a couple of weeks ago I had been feeling fine?

Once we got home I went back to bed. As long as I was lying down I was okay, but if I tried to get up I was dizzy. My vision was starting to go. I couldn't see if I tried to look directly in front of me. I could only see a little if I looked out through the sides of my eyes. Even that line of sight was diminishing. I was losing my eyesight and felt so helpless. I felt so alone. Even though I knew I had Mark and my family, this situation was mine alone. I needed to try to sort all this out. We didn't tell anyone what was going on except for those very close to us, and even then it was limited. It was for no other reason than we needed to know what was happening first. Some of my closest friends didn't know. I'm not sure if at that point I had even told my mother. It was a very confusing time for us.

At one point I was alone at home and had to take my medicine. I went downstairs to the kitchen where I knew the bottles were. I couldn't read what was written on the bottle and thought I knew which was which. I needed to take my vertigo medicine but by mistake took the sedative without knowing it. Later, I couldn't remember if I had to take the sedative or the vertigo medicine. I was so loopy from the extra sedative that I had taken and realized I had taken the wrong pill. It was scary how easily, when you're on all of those kinds of medications, you can mistakenly take the wrong ones and possibly overdose without knowing it. I was very careful after that. I didn't like taking pills to begin with. What a lonely feeling was filling my heart. How would I be able to take care of my kids in this condition? It wasn't safe for me to be in charge of anything at this point. I couldn't read. I couldn't even drive. I could do absolutely nothing except wait to find out what was causing all of this.

I was very sick in bed for weeks. My vision at times was almost gone. When I finally made it out of bed, I tried to watch T.V. but could only see it if I looked out of the side of my eye. If I tried to watch straight on, the screen was completely distorted or dark. I was still dizzy and my balance was completely off. I still couldn't feel the right side of my face and head. I was so fatigued.

It was the holiday season. I have always loved everything about Christmas. I loved decorating the house and getting a big Christmas tree. I managed to do all of it that year, but it was incredibly difficult. Trying to make everything look normal and manageable was quite a challenge for me. I still couldn't drive or see very well and there was a lot that needed to be done. To this day, I have no idea how it all got accomplished.

Up to this point in my life, I had been very self-sufficient. I'd never hesitate to help my family and friends, but I had a very hard time asking for help. It was hard for me to show any sign of weakness. It was a matter of too much pride, although I didn't know it at the time. I didn't tell anyone about what was happening unless is was absolutely necessary because I didn't want anyone's pity. Being the strong one was all I knew. I had always been the caretaker. So now the roles were different. I needed to be taken care of and I didn't know how to go about it.

Looking back, there is no doubt in my mind that if I had reached out for help it would have come from so many different directions. As I think about it now, it was another lesson I needed to learn. But it was one that was not an easy one. We are a product of what we think we know and who we think we have to be. This is not necessarily who we are. It is who we think others want us to be. How silly is that? If we just realize that all we have to do is come from our hearts and live in the moment at all times, our perceived stress would melt away. That's a lesson I desperately needed to learn.

CHAPTER 3

Wrong Answer

I was referred to a neurologist said to be the very best in Newport Beach. I had no idea what to expect or why I had to see him exactly. I had never been so scared or felt so alone in my life. It was a different loneliness. I was obviously completely out of commission, but had no way of putting aside the guilt that I was feeling for being sick. Guilt for all the trouble and disruption I was causing in my family's life, in particular, Mark's life. He was working so hard and now had to carry double duty. I was used to lifting up everyone else around me, but this time I was needing the lifting and I didn't know how to go about doing that. I needed to find out what was wrong with me and I had to get better for my husband and my little ones.

Mark drove me to the neurologist appointment. The office was very upscale and pleasant. It was obviously the office of a successful practice. We met with the doctor and talked about my symptoms. He suggested I do a spinal tap. I had heard those words before, but I really didn't know what they meant. Well, it wasn't pleasant. He had me lie on my side with my back toward him and he put a needle in my spine to take out fluid. At the time it made no sense to me. Why would he be taking fluid out of my spine? Today I know he was looking for protein in the fluid to see if he could detect signs of MS. Once done he sent me on my way to wait until he got the results of all the tests and MRI scans to determine what was wrong with me. At this point my eyesight was next to gone, my balance was still not good, I had no depth perception, and my face was still numb. Other symptoms came and went. I was so, so fatigued.

All I could do was wait to get some answers. Life was running along and I was not running with it. Other people were now taking my children to school and to their activities. The girls and I planned to go to our first tea together for our mother-daughter organization and I had to ask my mother-in-law to go with them because I couldn't go. I was starting to feel frustrated and sorry for myself, and for them. It is at these moments in life, when our bodies force us to stop and take stock, that we need to do so. We need to listen and pay attention, but we seldom do.

Finally, I had an appointment to go back to the neurologist to learn about my test results and his diagnosis. On our way up in the elevator, Mark said, "It's going to be fine." I desperately needed for that to be true. We walked into the doctor's office and sat down across from him. He seemed pleased. He had looked at all the tests and he said all the results were good. The MRI was normal. The spinal tap showed a slight something, but that he thought it may have been tainted in the lab. The rest of the tests were perfect. He believed my symptoms would go away and I would be like new in no time. This was coming from a very successful neurologist—a neurologist who was so successful he may have been too busy to take a look at the MRI. But at this point I didn't know that. All I knew was that the doctor said I was fine! Hallelujah! That is exactly what we wanted to hear. I was elated. We both walked out of there ecstatic at what we had been told. It was just a matter of waiting patiently for the symptoms to pass, and, in fact, I did begin to feel better. Not completely normal, but better. Christmas was coming and all would be well again.

I distinctly remember trying so hard to behave as if nothing was wrong. I was dizzy and off balance, but trying very hard to walk as if nothing was happening. My intention was to move through the holidays and never let on how awful I was feeling. I had to miss a couple of events at the beginning of the season simply because I couldn't get out of bed, but I was determined to try to make everything "normal" again. My feeling was that if I was determined enough, I would be able to get beyond it.

Christmas Eve came and we spent it with the whole family. It is one of my favorite times of year, but I was having a very hard time keeping it together and enjoying this one. I remember walking through the living room into the dining room and trying so hard to not let on that I was having difficulty keeping my balance. I thought I was being successful at hiding it. That is the only memory I have of that Christmas Eve—trying so hard to keep it together. My mother-in-law noticed what was happening to me. Although she didn't say anything that night, and she let the holidays pass before she approached me, she made it clear she wanted to discuss what was happening with me. It would be the last Christmas I would spend with my dad.

CHAPTER 4

The Diagnosis

My mother-in-law worked as a nurse for a great neurologist. After the holidays she tried to convince me to get a second opinion with him. I fought it. I was annoyed at the idea that there was a possibility I might not be fine. I already had the news I'd wanted. Why should I get a second opinion? I wanted so desperately to be fine, and the thought of anyone telling me any differently scared me.

Finally, after a few weeks of contemplation and stalling, I made an appointment to see her doctor. I was asked to bring all my tests and MRI scans. Once they were in my hands I never looked at them. As it turns out, the doctor my mother-in-law worked for was an MS specialist. He was the president of the Multiple Sclerosis Society and a leading authority in his field. He had dedicated his career and his life to helping people afflicted with this disease. Now mind you, I didn't know what his specialty was and to be quite honest had no awareness of MS at the time. My mother-in-law, on the other hand, knew a lot about MS and was recognizing what was happening to me.

The day came to see the doctor. My symptoms came and went. My vision was starting to come back, but I still couldn't see well and I had no real depth perception. My head and face were still numb. My balance was off and now I had a burning sensation in my ears. It was as if someone was putting a hot rod inside my ear canal. I felt weak and so, so fatigued. Pretending to feel well was getting harder and harder. As Mark and I drove to the doctor's, I had a knot in my stomach. I had no idea what he could possibly think I might have. I just knew that there was a possibility he might find something I didn't want to have.

We got to the building and checked in at the front desk. My mother-in-law was away at a conference, but everyone knew who I was and why I was there. We waited in the waiting room; the same waiting room I have been visiting since. Finally we went to the exam room. I gave the nurse my tests and MRI scans for Dr. Van De Noort to see. The waiting seemed like forever. Then the door to the room opened and in walked a little man with the kindest eyes and smile I had ever seen in a physician. He was older and slightly hunched as if he had spent many years looking into a microscope, over a patient, or reading medical research and charts at his desk. This was a man who had dedicated his life to his patients and it was palpable. He introduced himself and sat down on a chair positioned near me. Then he said something that would change my life forever. I can't remember the specifics, but it was something to the effect of: "I looked at your MRI and there is no doubt that you have Multiple Sclerosis."

I had no idea what Multiple Sclerosis was, but I was certain that it was not good. My mind rushed to try to retrieve anything I had ever heard or knew about those two words. All of this processed in the span of seconds, and with it an uncontrollable need to cry. And cry I did. He handed me a tissue and let me cry. Eventually he started talking in a gentle and soothing voice telling me that I didn't need to worry. That what was in store for me was a little help from a walking cane in a very distant future, in the same way most people would need it. The good news was that there was medicine now for MS and he recommended that I get on it right away. The lesions in my brain indicated that my MS was aggressive and that the sooner I got on the medicine the faster we could stop the progression of more lesions. Dr. Van De Noort insisted I not worry and that I was going to be fine. He and Dr. GT would be with me every step of the way. I would be very well taken care of, and so many other reassuring words I'm sure I haven't done justice here. He explained what MS was, but to be honest I don't remember that. I focused on some of what he said and let go of other things. His reassurance and strength would enable me to be strong. He gave me a short book on MS and a prescription for medicine.

I was in shock. I didn't know what MS was. I didn't know what all of this meant. Although Dr. Van De Noort said I was going to be fine, my gut feeling was that it wasn't going to be quite like that. Even though he was giving me encouraging words, I knew that unless the symptoms I was feeling went away, my life would never be the same again. But it is those words that gave me the spark of hope which I would need to try to get back to my old self. He set the tone, and that is why it's so important to have a doctor who is in your corner with an encouraging outlook. We will talk more about that later.

So now what? Would I ever drive again? Would I ever play tennis or ski again? What was going to happen to me? What was going to happen to my family? I had three kids who needed me. I had a husband who should have a healthy wife. I was stunned. I had known for months that there was something very wrong, but I wasn't prepared for this.

CHAPTER 5

Rock Bottom

The next morning I woke up and Mark was lying in bed next to me. Even though he wasn't saying anything, I knew he was awake. I didn't say anything either. I just wondered how he was feeling, and what he was thinking. I was afraid to ask... I lay there wondering what our life was going to be like. I loved him so much. We had already been through so much together. Our life was now starting to get easy, and we were enjoying this life we had built. He needed a wife who was healthy. I thought of my three babies. I wasn't sure how I was going to manage. My goodness, this was not something I had planned for. It's crazy how our lives can change in an instant.

That same day I got a call from one of my dearest friends. She wanted to take me out and meet with a couple other friends for dinner, one of whom also had MS. I didn't know it at the time, but their plan was to talk to me about having MS over dinner. The evening turned out to be nothing like that. We ate, drank wine, and talked and laughed for hours. The conversation never turned to what they had planned. That night I felt loved and protected. I felt as if I was in one of those old black and white movies where the wagons circle to protect themselves from the attack of the Indians as they cross the plains. These women were the wagons that circled around me and protected me from this hiccup in my life. They made me feel safe, even if only for a night. That's the power of love and friendship.

During the following months, only thoughts of the MS diagnosis filled my mind. Would I ever be able to think of anything else?! I was so sad. I was filled with self-pity and doubt. So, as it turned out, there was no pill

I could take. There was medicine though, and very good medicine. There was only one catch—it needed to be injected. Did I mention I was terrified of needles? This was going from bad to worse. Once a week I was going to have to have an injection. How was I going to do that?

Again, my mother-in-law came to my rescue and said she would train me in the proper way to inject. Instead of having a stranger teach me, she would do it. So we set up a time and date to meet at her house. We sat around a table in her family room and she explained the process very clearly to me. I understood, but still wondered how in the world I would be able to do it. I was deathly afraid of needles. The thought of them made me feel queasy. This was not going to be easy. It came time for me to do it to myself. They waited and waited and waited and waited for me to get up the courage to do it by myself, after practicing on other things. She finally offered to do it for me, but I took a very deep breath and finally after what must have seemed like hours, I did it. Crying the whole time. Unbelievable that I had been able to do that. Although I was scared beyond belief, in a strange way it was empowering for me. I knew then I would be able to do this. I did not want to depend on others if I could help it.

I was told to take an over the counter sleep aid so I would sleep through the side effects of the medicine. I did that and expected to sleep. I fell asleep, but a couple of hours later woke up aching and had what felt like a fever. My whole body was shaking. I felt like I had a horrible case of the flu. These were the side effects of the medicine. I was going to feel like this for 24 hours every time I took the medicine. It was unbelievable to me that this was going to be my reality once a week for the rest of my life. The next day I felt like I had been run over by a truck. Just add that to everything else that was happening to me. I was feeling sorry for myself now. This time period is fuzzy with just some very clear moments, like the first time I took my medicine. Injecting myself once a week became my new normal routine. At this point I wasn't sure what was going to happen to me. I was not telling many people what was going on. For whatever reason I wanted to keep it to myself. Perhaps I needed to fully understand it first. I didn't want to be defined by this disease, but I felt responsible to tell those who needed to know. I remember waking up and thinking "so I'm going to feel like this once a week for 24 hours the rest of my life."

I had volunteered to chair my daughter's graduation dance. The woman who was doing it with me was a new friend who I was getting to know through the activities at school. It was important that I tell her about my situation right away so she could find someone else to do this with her. We went to an event together and then had dinner. During dinner I told her what was happening and that I didn't know whether I could be of much help. She responded by saying that she didn't want to do it without me, that we would get through this together and that she would be there for me. This was the second time those around me seemed to have more faith in my recovery than I did. I was really stunned by how much love I was receiving. Was it possible for me to rise to their expectations? My husband kept saying I would be fine, and my kids still had no idea how bad the diagnosis really was. I wanted to keep it that way as long as I possibly could.

As I took the medicine I started feeling better. My vision returned to normal. The heat in my ears went away. The numbness in my head started fading. My depth perception started slowly coming back. Only my balance didn't seem to be getting better. As much as I hated taking the medicine, it was helping. I dreaded that one night a week when I took it. It was every Wednesday night like clockwork after dinner. For 24 hours after, I would be sick and then get better. It was definitely a love-hate relationship.

During this time I read everything I could on the subject of MS researching this mystery illness. As you may know by now, it's a fickle disease. The symptoms are different for everyone. There isn't one rule of thumb for the way it will progress. There is no rhyme or reason for why it behaves one way with one individual and another way with another. But in all of my research, one of the things that jumped out at me was the belief that stress was directly tied somehow to the aggravation of symptoms. In my case, I found this to be true. The numbness on my face had begun to decrease. My forehead and nose were no longer numb. The area around my right ear was no longer numb. But, something curious started happening. When I became stressed the numbness around my mouth and cheek became more pronounced and would start to spread. So, now I had a very physical gauge on my emotional status. There were times when I didn't realize I was getting stressed until the numbness started spreading.

This allowed me to figure out that I needed to manage my stress and any negative emotions. I had to find a way. I read in a book they gave me when I was diagnosed that yoga and Tai Chi possibly alleviated MS symptoms. My gym had yoga classes that coincided with the family's schedule going there. Things were lining up for me to do this, so I started taking yoga classes. I was very fortunate to find a good teacher. I attended the classes faithfully at least three times a week. Physically and mentally I was able to begin to acknowledge stressful situations without letting them take over me. My balance slowly came back physically, as well as emotionally. A whole new world was opening up thanks to yoga. I was able to ride a bike again—something I thought I would never do... And that was just the beginning. Not only can I ride a bike now, but I drive, play tennis, walk a few miles a day, practice and teach yoga. Do you remember that when I initially got sick I was trying to go skiing and couldn't? Well, I now can ski again. I can do all the things I did before getting sick, and more.

My mother got very ill at about the same time I found out I had MS. My father was also deteriorating physically rapidly, after being sick for many years, and passed away a couple of months after I was diagnosed. Talk about stress! It really was a very bleak time in my life. But because of the place I was in physically and mentally from the MS, I learned to flow with the reality that all of these events were out of my control and I had to let go… That doesn't mean that I wasn't sad about my father's death or terrified for what might happen to my mother; it just meant that they were painful events in my life that needed to be. It was necessary for me to feel the pain of my loss, but not perceive it as overwhelming. I've learned stress comes from the belief that we have some control over a situation. The reality is that life happens. I was learning that we have to take life as it is and acknowledge that life simply *is*. We can only change our thoughts and behavior, and in turn they will help us to change our physical reactions and emotional well-being. I'm talking about a mind-body connection that I've found, and want to help you find it too.

CHAPTER 6

The Light Switch Is Turned On

One night as I was taking my shot, maybe six or eight months into the process, I decided that I wasn't going to "hate" the medicine anymore. It was there to help me. And it *was* helping me. It was now going to be completely my ally. It had to be all or nothing for me. As I went through the process of filling the syringe with the vials that had to be mixed and injecting, all I kept thinking was that this helped me and was good for me. I would no longer see it as a pain, but rather a blessing. I visualized the medicine as little soldiers going into my body to heal me. I visualized it going to my brain and flowing throughout my whole body. When I finished the process, I thanked it for helping me. I thanked it for being available to me and for its ability to heal me. That night I slept through the night with no flu symptoms. The next day I woke up and had no flu symptoms and none for the rest of the day. I felt strong and vibrant. I had so much energy for the first time since the diagnosis, and I felt happy. I was actually looking forward to the next shot. When the next Wednesday came I followed the same process and, like magic, I slept through the night again and woke up feeling strong! Every Wednesday thereafter was to be the same. It was as if the shots were now charged with energy. They made me feel strong. I felt so empowered, and very lucky.

This was the beginning of a very serious experience with how strong my mind could be in this process. It was amazing to me that a shift in my attitude could do this. The only thing that had changed was how I chose to perceive my relationship with my medicine. I was in no way experienced with this. I had no special abilities and no idea that it would be possible.

However, I did have a fierce determination to get better. I had and continue to have a burning desire to figure out how and why this was happening to me. Not only how or why, but how to move beyond it and get better. That was the beginning of remarkable happenings in my life.

My vision was back. My balance wasn't quite there, but I was on my way to feeling better. I could drive again. I was driving in my car and turned on the CD player. In it was a cd Mark had been playing while driving my car and out of curiosity I decided to listen to it. It was one of about a dozen CD's in a series on the power of positive thinking by guest speakers for Anthony Robbins. This particular one was Deepak Chopra. The only thing I knew of Deepak Chopra then was that he was a little "out there." Not sure how I had come to that conclusion, but I knew that his ideas were suppose to be very "new age," even though I had never taken the time to really listen to anything he had to say. This time I did listen, and I can't tell you why. What I heard was so incredible to me that there was no doubt in my mind that I was meant to hear it. Deepak Chopra was talking about the ability of the body to heal itself. That our cells renewed themselves every few weeks and whether they were healthy or not when they renewed was dependent on our thoughts. If we were to change our signals/thoughts we sent to our brains with positive healing thoughts, we could shift the body into health. He said much more, but this is what I walked away with. He also talked about having a center in Massachusetts. When I heard that, I decided I needed to go there to see him. I couldn't contain myself or the excitement of what was happening. Never in my life had I thought this could be possible, but I was starting to live it…

I reached my office and told Mark what I had heard and told him I wanted to go to see Dr. Chopra. We jumped on the computer, researched him and as it turned out, he had moved his center to La Jolla, California, which was about an hour and a half away from me. I couldn't believe it! I got on the phone and made an appointment to go to the center for a full work-up.

A week later I was driving to La Jolla for a 7:00 a.m. appointment. This was my first long drive by myself since I had been diagnosed. I had no idea what to expect, but this was the beginning of a series of events that would shape the course of my life. Dr. Chopra wasn't there to see me, but his partner, Dr. Simon, was. Dr. Simon happened to be a neurologist by profession and now he practiced mind-body medicine at the center. We talked and he examined me. I was introduced to the science of Ayurveda and was given recommendations specific to my body. The importance of what I ate was stressed. This included yellow, orange and red fruits and vegetables. He recommended whole foods rather than processed foods, along with other food suggestions specific to my mind and body type. He also introduced the importance of self-care. This included self-massage and attention to my body to create a space for self-healing and balance. I remember asking him if he thought I would get better. He looked at me and said, simply, "Yes." He said I would be better once my body was brought back to balance and I followed their suggestions. This was the second doctor who told me I would be fine. I can't stress enough how important that was in the process of my healing. At no point did I hear from my doctors that I would not be well.

Once finished with the medical work-up I was introduced to a man to learn meditation. He took me into a small room and I sat on a chair across from him. He talked to me about meditation, the process of meditating, and taught me how to meditate with focus on breath and a mantra. Let me just say, that up until that point, I thought this kind of stuff was way too "out there" and just plain weird. As far as I was concerned this kind of thing was a crock. But what did I have to lose? Then I fell, and I mean fell, into a deep meditation without realizing it was happening. It was absolutely incredible. All the notions I had on the subject went out the window as I realized the power of what I was learning. An hour and a half later I came out of my session with him feeling calm and refreshed, and with an incredible sense of peace.

I was taken to a dining room for lunch after meditation. The food was vegetarian and different from how I normally ate, but it was delicious. It was a leisurely, relaxed lunch in a very serene environment. Other people joined me. A couple of them were nurses who were learning techniques to help patients relax and heal. They practiced Western medicine in a conventional hospital, but had been finding that these techniques were very valuable to the patients they saw. Nothing "weird" about them. I was still a little skeptical about all of this, in spite of how good I was feeling.

Next I was taken to a room for massage. I loved massages, but I had never looked at massage as a healing tool. I thought of them as a way of indulging myself. That all changed after that day. I was taken to a typical quiet, tranquil massage room. I was given two different types of massage, both Ayurvedic, and I experienced a whole new level of ease and relaxation. It felt like it was happening at a cellular level and was unlike anything I had ever experienced before. During the first massage they dripped hot oil on my forehead and throughout my head. When I read the description of that massage before going there, I thought it was going to be a torture. Little did I know the incredible effects it would have on me. The second one was given by two people simultaneously. During that hour I felt as if I was suspended in a lightness like I had never experienced before. Dripping in oil and feeling a level of well-being that is indescribable; the sessions ended three hours later. I sat for some time and let the oils stay on my skin before showering. The whole experience was settling into my body, but it was also being digested by my nervous system and my brain. Never had I experienced anything like that. Healing was taking on a whole new meaning at a whole new level. My body was so receptive to this healing process.

I ended my day at the Chopra Center with a yoga class. I was already familiar with yoga, but this class was different from what I had been taking at my gym. The class at the gym was helping me physically to get my balance back. It had definitely helped me regain most of it, but this yoga class took it a step further. In this class I caught a glimpse of yoga in its original form. It prepared me for the class I would eventually find that would lead me to total well-being.

As I drove home that day I felt hopeful and certain that there was more to healing. My body and my mind felt more relaxed and balanced than they had in a very, very long time. I realized I was onto something here. There really was hope, and I knew I would get better. I didn't necessarily know how this was to happen, but I was certain it would. I felt a fire ignite in me. Faith was now my weapon of choice. As I drove home, I realized that the debilitating fatigue that had become my day-to-day reality had been replaced by relaxation and a sense of incredible well-being. The drive home in the early evening along the coast of California, with the ocean on my left, was one of joy and excitement for the possibilities of what was happening to me. My intuition told me I was exactly where I needed to be at that point in time. As strange as all of this was to me, it felt right.

CHAPTER 7

Yoga Shmoga

When I got home I told Mark all about my incredible day. The look of hope on his face mirrored how I was feeling inside. It really was a very strange and quick turn of events for us. You must understand, this was all very bizarre to us. I had grown up with a mother who went to holistic doctors, but to me all of it was hocus-pocus. Mark listened to motivational recordings, but for motivational purposes, certainly not for any kind of healing. That his CD was in my car at that point in time for me, was quite remarkable and I was well aware of that.

I continued to go to my yoga classes at my gym and continued to get more of my balance back, but I really wanted to find something like I had found at the Chopra Center. I couldn't explain at the time what that was, but I knew that it was out there for me. One day shortly after, out of the blue, without knowing anything about my MS diagnosis, my friend Divya asked if I was taking yoga. She is from India and told me that I needed to go to her yoga class. She insisted that it was the best class around with no comparison. I nodded and humored her by telling her I would go some time, but at that time I really had no intention of going. Mind you, it makes no sense to me now that I didn't jump at that opportunity. It took me about six months before I finally agreed to go. The class was about 30 miles from my home on Wednesday evenings. Very inconvenient, but I could drive now so I could do it. Divya and I were going to meet at the class.

Wednesday came and at 6:00 p.m. I left my house to be at the class by 7:00 p.m. I knew very little about Indian culture. As a child I travelled often by myself flying from Venezuela to California. My parents were divorced and I lived with my mother in Venezuela and would visit my dad in California in the summers. That was during the late 60s and throughout the 70s. During the late 60s and early 70s at the airports there were always young women and men with flowers trying to pin them on you and asking for donations. They were all part of the Hare Krishna movement of that time, and they scared me. They all seemed to have a strange look in their eyes and a strange smile. Mind you, this is the perspective of a little girl who had no idea what it was all about, but it made a lasting impression. I give you this background so that you know just how ignorant I was and how little I knew about the culture. That I was taking yoga was a miracle in itself.

I drove up to the parking lot of the yoga class and it was fairly empty. My friend wasn't there yet and I was one of the first to arrive so I found a spot near the back. That was usually my seat of choice no matter where I went. The class wouldn't be starting for 20 minutes but I was glad to be there and to be able to settle in before it began. The room was in a community center. It was modern and very big. I could see where it could be partitioned into two rooms. I wasn't used to being in such a large room for yoga. I was thinking that there would be plenty of room for anyone who came. Pretty soon the class started filling up and my friend was nowhere to be seen. The room filled up, the doors closed, and I realized I was the only American in the room. Not only was I the only American in the room, but even though the class was crowded, there was a very nice big space all around me. I was definitely the stranger in the class, or maybe it was my perception of what was happening. In any case, it didn't deter me. I was there to find out what this was all about, although I'll admit I was ready to be skeptical. I liked the class I was taking at my private gym. This class was in a community center. Not very fancy and definitely not very spiritual in surroundings. So much for insight. My ignorance and expectation of how I thought things should be was jading my perception. I was totally out of my element. Since being sick, that seemed to be the running theme in my life. The rug had been pulled out from under me and in almost all parts of my life I was feeling uncertain. But I was putting up a good front. I had decided to overcome whatever was happening to me, but wasn't sure whether I'd succeed. Honestly, I just didn't see that I had a choice. I had to get well. I just wanted to be there for my kids and my family. I was ready to try anything.

As I sat there with my eyes closed and my thoughts racing through my head, there was movement at the front of the class. A thin man with silver hair and a very straight posture was at the front of the class and he began chanting. I later found out it was a prayer for peace in Sanskrit, but at the time I realized this was a far cry from the yoga classes I was used to. Although my yoga teacher at my gym used different words for the postures, I really had no idea what language it was. I just hadn't gotten that far yet. Once that was over he translated the prayer into English and welcomed us all. He taught for the next hour and a half. I had some difficulty understanding him because he had a very heavy accent, but I knew most of the poses as I watched and followed along. At the end, the meditation was quite good. I left thinking that the class was good, but I couldn't really understand why Divya raved about it. Not only that, she never showed up to her amazing class!

The following week I agreed to meet her there again and really give the class a fair chance. Again, I got there early, settled in as people filled the class and was given a very nice space all around me, despite how crowded the class was. Again, Divya never showed up and the same gentleman taught the class. It was a very pleasant class, but I wasn't sure it was worth driving 45 minutes in traffic for it. I went back and forth on whether I would go back and again Divya convinced me to go, telling me she would meet me there this third time for sure. I can't explain why, but I decided to give the class a third chance.

Again, I got there early, found myself a spot and waited for Divya to arrive and for class to begin. I was in the back, in the last row. The door was behind me to the right, and the same gentleman who taught the last two classes was also there. I had my eyes closed and was sitting silently when I felt an energy come behind me and to my left. I didn't hear anything I just felt it. I opened my eyes and saw a man I had never seen before. He had silver hair and a walk that was more like gliding than walking. A very strong figure, he reminded me of a lion. He was wearing white pants and a white tunic pressed so immaculately it drew my attention. He went toward the front of the class and sat on the ground on a piece of cloth. I then realized who Divya had been talking about. The teacher she had been telling me about was this man, not the one I had been following the previous two weeks. That night was a yoga class like I had never experienced before. For two hours I listened and followed his instructions. He had an accent, but spoke very clearly with a deep, beautiful, soothing voice. His vocabulary was extensive and precise. As he spoke he began addressing some of the issues that had been in my heart and on my mind. I couldn't believe that I was being given insight to questions that he could never have known I had. I hated to see the class end. What an experience that was. Still Divya was a no-show. But now it didn't matter. I completely understood what she meant. This class was a gift.

I kept going to the class every Wednesday. It was my space in the middle of the week to an amazing world where I was on a single journey, but unafraid, and all of my questions were being addressed. Quite a remarkable experience. Now, that's not to say that the cynic in me was not a little disconcerted by all of it. But my heart was so sure that this was where I needed to be. Every Wednesday from then on I was there early and ready to receive. It felt good to be alone on this path. It felt right to be alone. Only I could understand what was happening to me. There was no need to try to explain or chat because I knew no one there. It felt so good to just be. The only time I spoke was when walking out of class; then I would thank the teacher and leave.

Although I was enjoying my new yoga classes, I still had questions as to whether I should start practicing Tai Chi or continue only with yoga. I was ready to try any and everything I possibly could to get better. So I was tirelessly exploring what would be the best for my situation. I had no idea about all of this, but knew someone who practiced both. He was a young American guy who was a friend of the family. We had known him for years, but we were not close. My husband contacted him to get more information on the different practices he practiced and to try to decide what to do. When I started telling him I was practicing yoga he explained the benefits of both. I then told him I had found a new class I was really interested in but not sure about. Being a longtime dedicated practitioner, I figured he could shed some light on this. We discussed the style and type of class it was. When I told him whom I was taking the class from he said, "You are in very good hands. Soneji's the real thing. I know him very well." He suggested I stay in that class and learn all I could from him, and to stop looking elsewhere. Needless to say I was blown away. That was not at all what I expected. Of all the people he could have known, how in the world did he know my teacher? But how glad I am at the outcome.

That gave me more confidence in my choice. Although I was seeing the results of practicing yoga, I was very cautious and maybe a little suspicious of all of this *mumbo jumbo.* I never spoke to anyone in the class, including the teacher. I would thank him at the end of class and go home. But, the effect this class was having on me was indescribable. Things in me were settling in, settling down, and balance was coming back to my body. At this point I was still taking my medicine, and as a matter of fact, I think I was taking it on Wednesday nights after class.

CHAPTER 8

Letting Go

After a year of going religiously to class every Wednesday evening, I called Soneji to make an appointment to talk to him. He always said in class that for any questions he was always available by appointment. I had finally reached a point where my cynicism had died down and I wanted to talk to him to see what he could tell me about my MS. He agreed to meet with me a few days later. Notice that I called it "my MS." That is how I thought of it. I hadn't begun to let it go.

I reached Soneji's house in the morning, knocked on the door and waited. He opened the door and asked me to come in. We sat in his living room and I told him my story. He suggested a couple of breathing/pranayama techniques to do and asked me to continue going to class. Then he said, "Let's have something to eat." I was struck by his matter of fact demeanor, his kindness and selflessness. I'm not sure that I had ever met anyone like him. Even though I said I couldn't have anything to eat, he wouldn't take *no* for an answer. He asked me if I liked carrots and he proceeded to make fresh carrot juice and fill a bowl with nuts. As we ate, he asked me what I normally ate for breakfast. I told the truth. My preference was a bagel with cream cheese and coffee with cream. As I write this, I'm so fully aware of how bad my choice of breakfast was for me—someone specifically allergic to wheat. No wonder my body was going haywire. Well, he laughed and said that we all had our preferences and that he was sure I must enjoy my bagels. No judgment there. How unusual that was. How unusual this man was.

We finished breakfast. I ate to be polite, but ultimately wound up enjoying it. More than what we ate, I enjoyed the way in which we ate. It was calm and serene. He and I were very relaxed and everything took place in a slow, easy manner. That was not something I was use to. I thanked him and left feeling light and healthy. That hour with Soneji had been absolutely free of stress and pressure of any kind, and the effect it had on me was that of lightness. I could feel the difference in my body—but more than my body, my mind.

Wednesdays came and Wednesdays went and unless I was on vacation, I was in class, sitting in the back of the room. I was enjoying every moment and wishing they never ended. Wednesdays weren't enough for me. I needed more, but I needed more on my own. I needed to give myself the time to understand what it was all about. My feeling was that this was something I needed to look into deeper, not just follow. So, beyond the class, I started taking what I was learning and doing it at home. The solitude of this practice was interesting and comforting for me. I began to study the effect of certain postures on my body. Every time it was different. Every day, seemingly the same on the outside, was a new adventure with my body and my mind. I practiced the breathing techniques and became so intimately involved in the process. I was in awe of this amazing body and how it worked. The incredible power and energy of my breath was humbling and my gratitude and love for that process began to grow. My understanding of the effect of my breath on my health, on my body and on my mind was such an "aha" moment for me. It is so essential it's nearly indescribable. Then came the meditations.

I don't remember exactly how it happened, it just did. I began spending more time in silence. I began loving my time in silence. There again, every time is different. It was a joy to know that every time I sat down to meditate it would be a different adventure for me.

I want to share this quote with you: "Please tell not the Universe that my difficulties are bigger, please tell the difficulties my Universe is bigger." "My" universe had grown exponentially since I had become sick and the illness was having less and less of an impact. It had gone from "my" MS to simply MS. I no longer identified with it. The possibilities of what life had to offer and what I had to offer to life were shifting. I had so many questions, yet all were being answered and I was open to the answers. I don't believe in coincidences. I believe that this man was put in my path to help me and he has indeed done that. I also believe he was put in my path so that I can help others. And now, after many, many years of study and practice, I can pass along some of what I've learned from him and others along the way to healing. There is no question in my mind that it has been through these processes that I have been able not only to regain my old self, but have turned into a new improved self, physically, mentally, as well as spiritually. I must emphasize that I have no hidden talents or tools that aren't accessible to everyone. What has happened has been through a process of self-love and self-care that had been forgotten somewhere along the way. We think that always putting others before us is *the* giving, altruistic way. The reality is that before we can give, we have to have something to give. If we don't nurture and recharge ourselves we won't have anything left to give. We must be clear in the fact that we have to be true to our paths. We must live in such a way that what we think, say, and do are in alignment. I may not have the ideal job, but I am so lucky that I have the health to go to work. What I am trying to tell you is, that we must create the world we want, for us and for our loved ones. We must be involved in the things we truly love in our spare time, not those that we think are what others want us to be involved. We have a choice. We must respect our own choices and, in doing so, health and well being will follow because the signals we are sending to our bodies are those of joy and fulfillment rather than misery and discontent.

By the way, I'm still waiting for my friend Divya to show up to class. She had no idea I was sick. I believe that she may still not know what was happening to me at that time. That makes it even more wonderful. Every so often, when I see her I tell her how grateful I am to her for having introduced me to Soneji's yoga class. She has no idea the depth of my gratitude. She very well may have saved my life.

I think my life was always this way, but I didn't listen well enough. Now, I was becoming more aware. The way things were presenting themselves really was nothing short of miraculous. Mark had a very bad pain in his shoulder and a friend of ours suggested he go to her acupuncturist. In a few weeks, the acupuncturist had been able to solve a problem her husband had for many years, and had been able to help her as well. So Mark went and, sure enough, the pain was resolved. While he was there he told the doctor that I had MS and asked if he thought he could help. He told him he wouldn't know until he saw me and even then he couldn't guarantee anything. As much as I was afraid of needles, I had a very good feeling about it. I made an appointment and went to see Dr. Lee. We talked and he asked me all sorts of questions, which covered personality, habits and eating patterns. He looked at my eyes. He made me stick out my tongue and show it to him, and he took my pulse in both arms. Then he said, "I think I can help you. Don't worry, you will be okay." I was feeling all right, but I wanted to be even better. So I began going to the acupuncturist every week. Dr. Lee would begin with me at 9:00 a.m. and end at around 1:00 p.m., every Sunday for a little over a year. He would look at my tongue, take my pulse, and then put together herbs for my tea for that week. Then he would have me lie down on my back and would give me about 20 minutes to relax. He would place needles all over the front of my body. During this process, I would keep my eyes closed because I couldn't look at the needles. Then he would leave and I would lie there for 20 minutes or so by myself. I decided that I would take that time to meditate. I would mindfully try to help in my healing process. I would visualize and meditate the whole time. He would then come in to remove the needles and I would relax some more. Then I would lie on my stomach and he would put the needles into the back side of me. Again, I would take the time to meditate and focus to try to help him heal me. So for over a year, I would spend about two hours every Sunday meditating in the name of wellness.

One day, about 15 months after beginning with him, Dr. Lee said to me, "Margie, it's time for you to have an MRI." Although I had never seen my prior MRI's, I knew I had lesions in my brain. When I started my process with Dr. Lee I made the decision to stop taking my medicine. My health was stable, the medicine had done its job in bringing me back to health, but I was ready to take the next step. The next step meant having faith that between the yoga practice and the acupuncture I would be able to bring my body back to balance and health without the medicine. Now it was time to see what happened.

CHAPTER 9

Face to Face With My MRI

A month later I was in a tube having another MRI. Many thoughts were going through my head. Then it dawned on me how much I had changed over the years. For the first MRI they gave me a sedative to help me cope with my claustrophobia. The following MRI's weren't quite as bad, but definitely still unpleasant experiences. This time, my fear was not in the physical aspect of the MRI. Quite the contrary. I was very comfortable with the whole situation. My fears were of the result. How much I had overcome without knowing it! After it was over, I was still amazed at how easy the whole process had been for me in comparison.

The call came… I distinctly remember answering the phone in the kitchen. Dr. GT had the results of the MRI. She sounded excited and happy! She wanted to see me and wanted me to bring all my other MRI's with me. The results of my MRI were excellent! I felt this huge sense of relief when I heard those words. I had acted on faith with the hope that I was doing the right thing, but knowing that the possibility of it being quite the opposite was always there. So I went for my appointment with all the MRI scans in my hands. She posted them in order in front of me so I could see them. I didn't want to look. I had never seen the MRI's. As illogical as I may sound, in my mind, if I didn't see it, the damage wasn't there. I know it makes no sense, but that is how I was able to cope with what was happening to me. I started crying, saying I didn't want to look and Dr. GT finally said, "You have to look. You have to see it." She had never forced anything on me. She had always encouraged me and allowed me to seek my health. So I looked. In the most recent MRI all the lesions were gone. Only one small spot was left. The reality of this was incredible. As I'm writing this I want to cry because it was such an overwhelming moment. There are no words to describe the gratitude I felt in that moment to know my health, and my life, was officially returning to me 7 years after the diagnosis.

Let me take a moment to clarify a few things. I am not sharing this part of my story to persuade you to stop taking medicine. Quite the contrary. The medicine is what brought me back to health in order for me to even think of attempting taking a solely holistic route. I believe that the medicine has its place. But I *do* believe that you can help yourself by helping the medicine. You can help yourself by going to the source of what made you sick in the first place. We are so fortunate to have medicine for this disease, but go beyond that to the reason you became sick in the first place. In seeking out the origin, you will be able to heal.

CHAPTER 10

For You

After all these years of seeking, I am very healthy. So healthy that my doctors are amazed. I walk 2-3 miles a day and I teach two hours of yoga twice a week. In between, there is some stand-up paddling and anything else that piques my interest. In 2013, I went to Tibet with my 17 year old son. We began in Kathmandu, Nepal and then went into Tibet. We were with 48 other people from 14 different countries. As we made our way to our final destination we trekked the Himalayas; saw incredible sights and befriended people without knowing their language. We shared one common denominator—our humanity, our love. There was no doubt that in order to be there we were opening up and surrendering to that which guides us. We bathed in the highest lake in the world, with maybe some of the coldest water...

Our ultimate destination was Mount Kailash. We hiked the perimeter of the peak for three days at an altitude of about 18,000+ feet. The weather would change from one moment to the next. It went from sunny and hot to rain and hail in an instant. This may be one of the most difficult things I've ever done, but at the same time the best thing I have ever done. By the end we were all a family. It was an incredible journey I would have never imagined taking before becoming sick with MS. I felt a huge release of fear and an infinite amount of gratitude for the ability to experience it.

I am in a place of gratitude. I am in a place of ease. I am in a place of harmony. I am in a place of balance. I am in a place of love. Would I have been in this place if my life had been different? I don't think so. I was so wrapped up in being who I thought other people wanted or needed me to be that somewhere along the way I forgot about myself. It's easy to do. Even now I have to check on myself to avoid falling back into those old patterns.

A couple of years ago, I was helping my son's theater class with a fundraiser. I needed to pick up plates and utensils for a couple hundred people. I also had to pick up a host of other things from quite a few different stores. My cellphone kept ringing with questions that needed to be answered and I had to go to work that afternoon before heading to the fundraiser at 5:00 p.m. That morning I taught yoga and wasn't able to get going on all of these errands until close to 11:30 a.m. So I was definitely rushing and a little frantic. As I was driving in the middle of all of this, I realized how tense I was. My back was stiff, my jaw was clenched, and every part of my body was tight. Not only that, my mind was racing in a way that it had not raced for many, many years. To be specific, it had not raced like that since 1998. I pulled into a driveway, and stopped the car. It hit me like a ton of bricks. This is how I had been feeling all the time when I got sick. It dawned on me that this is what my life had been like. I felt an overwhelming sadness for that woman who I had been all those years ago. No wonder I got sick. It was quite an eye-opening moment. I knew what my life had been like, but I had not experienced it from my new perspective. I felt sorry for the old me. I wanted to hug the old me and love me for how far I had come. Needless to say, I shifted my attitude. I did everything that I needed to do with the awareness that it would all get done without having to feel frantic. I was grateful that at this point in my life I could do it!

Originally this first half was not going to be written . To be honest, I didn't like to think about that time in my life when I was so sick. I wasn't sure that I would remember much of it if I tried. I was afraid to dig too deeply. Maybe you wouldn't be interested in listening to what had happened to me anyway. Then as I started writing about my experience something started happening. I realized that maybe my daughter was right. Maybe it is necessary for you to hear about my journey because it's what *you* are going through. Maybe, just maybe, you will understand the importance of this for you.

The sole reason this book has been written is to help you. I believe the reason I got sick in the first place was so that I could help you. It has become my life's mission to help others going through the journey with illness. My intention is for you to access the part of you that will help you heal. Access that part of you which is excited about life. Access that part of you that recognizes love is who you are. Recognize that it's in that love that you will heal. You must love yourself deeply and unconditionally to bring your body back to harmony and wellness.

The second part of this book will tell you how. But more importantly than that, listen to yourself and what you need, at all times coming from a place of love. No one knows better than you do. Allow your heart to speak to you. I am very conscious of why I am this healthy. It's taken hard work and determination. It's taken letting go of fears and tears. But most importantly, it's taken faith without a shadow of a doubt that I could do it. So can you.

CHAPTER 11

First Things First

Before we go any further we have to talk about this *dis-ease* that you have and how you really feel about it. I know you are thinking that it's obvious how you feel about it, but is it? Before you became sick, were there times when you didn't want to do all the things you had committed to doing? Have there been any times when you wished you had an excuse to get out of something? And lastly, now that you're sick have you ever used the dis-ease as an excuse to not do something? We spend our lives racing through life, I know I did. In the back of your mind was there that awareness that you were overstretched and didn't know what to do about it? We fill every moment because we think that is what is expected of us. The only time we stop or slow down is when we are forced to.

Well, our bodies force us to stop. In their love for us, they have brought us to a complete halt because what we were doing was hurting us. We are being protected by our bodies because we have forced and pushed them so far, so fast, and so hard that there was no time given to self-love. Be very honest with yourself in answering these questions because they're important to your recovery. There is no room for judgment or reprimands; there is only room for awareness and acceptance. There is only room for a new awakening. In the same way your body has stopped you, it can help you heal once you have become aware of the ability to do so, and if you do it with the love and kindness it needs. Help yourself heal with the same compassion you would have for a child who needs nurturing and love. Allow yourself to love you and help yourself come back to harmony. In order to get better you have to be one hundred percent committed and willing to heal. You have to want this with every cell of your body. You have to want this more than you have ever wanted anything in your life. Then you can go forward knowing that whatever the past was, is in the past and what is ahead of you is only healing and passion for life. A fervent desire to have a full, healthy life. Then we can take the steps to do so.

First of all, I want to make sure that you have chosen a doctor who is a specialist in MS. Not only a specialist, but sensitive enough and positive enough to know that this is a disease that can disappear as easily as it came. The reality is that he or she really doesn't know whether it will get a lot worse, or just simply stay the same or go away. You may think that is a horrible thought, but it's a beautiful and encouraging thought. It gives us the room to try to figure out how we can make ourselves better. There is hope. You will definitely need a doctor in your corner that sees a good future and helps you to believe in it too, and not one who will tell you, and I am quoting a friend's doctor, to "go pick out a wheel chair." NO! You absolutely cannot think that it will be that way! So, Step 1 is to research and choose a doctor who will be a positive influence in your life. This is *your* life. You are not just a number or a statistic. Pick a doctor who will hope and be positive with you! This will be a very important person in your life. If you now have a doctor and it's all doom and gloom, change doctors! Don't be intimidated. It could be the most important choice you make along your journey back to health. Pick someone you will look forward to seeing at every appointment. This person is going to be your partner for a long time. Even after you are well, chances are you will continue to see them, just as a precaution.

We are so fortunate that there is medication now available for us. Had we been diagnosed before there was any treatment, we wouldn't be so lucky. I began taking my medicine right away. I learned to inject myself. I have to tell you that I think that is one of the hardest things I have had to face. I am still deathly afraid of needles, but for six years they became my reality. I got pretty good at injecting despite myself. The medicine made all the difference for me. It made me feel strong, my vision went back to normal, my balance returned. The fatigue was still there, but not as severe. Now, I don't experience fatigue at all. I get tired just as anyone would, but it is definitely a normal sense of tiredness. Initially I had awful flu-like symptoms for 24 hours after I would take the medicine. It would put me out of commission for a day or two after. But truly, once I set my mind to make it my ally, the symptoms stopped. I actually started feeling energized by the shot. I would imagine that I was injecting an army of healers into my body. I would give thanks for the ability to do this, as I was doing it. Mind you, I'm still not thrilled about having to do it, but I knew and still know how much it has helped me overcome my MS symptoms. So let me be clear in that you know how important I think it is to use what Western modern medicine has to offer us. The medication will alleviate the symptoms the disease is causing.

Once that is under way and under control, then I believe it is important to overcome the disease using alternative methods. Those will be the ones that will take care of the reason we became ill to begin with. We want to go to the root of the problem. Why the disease in the first place? Yes, we want to get rid of the symptoms, but if we can get rid of the reason for those symptoms in the first place, then balance and health for the body can be achieved.

Shortly after finding out I had MS, someone I knew told me I should read a book she said had changed her life. I would like to now pass this gift on to you. It was the beginning of many such gifts for me. The title of the book is *You Can Heal Your Life* by Louise Hay. One of the most amazing earth shattering events in my life was the day I opened this book. I read it through once and read it again and still read it at least twice a year. Then after seeing the changes taking place in my own life I proceeded to buy a copy of it for everyone I thought would be open to it and would benefit from it. I can't stress enough how important it is that you read this book and assimilate what is says as much as you can. It has changed my life and the lives of many people I know. It will change your life too. But you can't stop there. That is just the beginning of a wonderful life ahead of you.

In my search for self-healing I have come to know a lot of different avenues and roads that I can take. I've only chosen to take the few that my gut told me were right for me. Not all sounded like they were the right things for me to do. My doctor gave me a book to read on MS that first day I saw him. Within that book there was a very short paragraph which said yoga seemed to relieve some of the symptoms in some people. That sounded like just what was necessary for me! I took up yoga and have not let it go since. There is definitely a connection between the healing that is taking place in my body and practicing yoga. I can imagine how many things come to mind when you hear the word *yogi*. It doesn't mean that I have gone to a far away place and live as a monk or stand on my head. I am still happily married and have now three amazing grown kids who are thriving with a healthy mother. It means that I have become a happier and more grateful person than I ever imagined I could be. I'm grateful? Am I kidding…? Now you really think I'm a nut. How can I say I'm grateful when I have been told I have MS? Well, the truth of the matter is, that is the way my life has developed. I have stopped going through the motions in my life. I now live as much as possible, in the moment. I continue to plan for the future, but I have a need to live in the *now*. I am blessed in that I am back to "normal." My balance is back. I went skiing and couldn't believe that I could actually go down the intermediate runs. I can play tennis and drive. These and more are things I thought I'd never do again. That is the gift of yoga and MS in my life. Through the practice of yoga I have learned to minimize the impact of stress in my life. It is acknowledged in the medical community that there is a connection between stress and MS symptoms. I believe that stress is a trigger for MS. So, I also believe that if you reduce your level of stress, you can reverse the damage done and become more healthy and whole. I believe that there is undoubtedly a mind-body connection. I didn't always think this way. Until I had to try to help myself heal, I thought this type of thinking was a bunch of new wave hogwash. I have since changed my mind. I wish I had known how to balance my mind and my body many years ago, but it's better late than never. Please remember this: it's *never* too late. The second part and probably the most important part of this book will address yoga. There are certain postures most beneficial in alleviating MS symptoms. That's not to say you can't practice some of the other postures as well. You don't have to be flexible to practice yoga. You do as much as your body allows you to do. With time, it will become more flexible. The harder it is to do, the more you should do it. It simply means that that part of your body has become rigid and needs to be loosened—but always without pain. For those who physically can't do some of the practices it is important you do them mentally. Visualize them and go through the postures and breathing with eyes closed. As strange as that may sound to you, you will be surprised by the results. You will also learn proper breathing and the importance of breath. And the final gift will be suggestions for meditation. The meditation is very important to lower your stress. I have found my teacher who has guided me through my yogic process. His wisdom as a teacher of yoga is filled with tremendous knowledge and love. I will be guiding you and will give you the benefits of his wisdom.

MS affects our nervous system, and the largest part of our nerve endings are on our skin. This is among the reasons massage is very effective in lowering stress levels. The importance of being touched cannot be overlooked. It is of huge importance in our case. Besides being very relaxing, it is also a healing process. Again a person with an amazing power to help heal through massage was put in my path. This has been integrated into my life as part of a health support system. As she puts it, "The healing is not being done by me, I am facilitating your body to heal through the process." The bottom line is that it has helped incredibly. Of course, I believe in the healing power of acupuncture. You need to use all the tools at your disposal to help bring balance and health to your body and mind.

So, let's begin the healing process.

CHAPTER 12

Change in Lifestyle

Nutrition

A change in lifestyle needs to be all encompassing. Let's start with nutrition.

It's important that you be aware of the effects that certain foods and chemicals have on your body. So I will begin with what I believe you should not eat.

Here is the list:

1. Absolutely no artificial sweeteners of any kind, including agave. Most agave is highly processed and therefore has lost any beneficial properties it had in the first place. No diet drinks or diet foods.
2. No hydrogenated oils of any kind. You will find these in many, many processed foods. Check the labels.
3. No processed foods. If it comes in a box or a bag, try to avoid it. Avoid frozen dinners, and any meals that have been pre-made and ready-to-eat. Avoid meals that are made and packaged for readiness in serving. Try to eat fresh food.
4. No artificial colors or flavorings. You will find these in processed foods.
5. No wheat. Most pastas, crackers and cookies contain wheat. There are many processed foods that do too. You can substitute them with those made from rice, or other grains.
6. No grains containing gluten, such as wheat and rye.

7. Avoid all refined sugar. This includes refined honey. Refined honey is honey that has lost all its healing properties and is converted into sugar through a heating process. Instead, choose raw honey.
8. Keep dairy intake to a minimum.

Take a trash bag and go through your cupboards and refrigerator. Take everything which is on the list above and put it in the bag. Look at the ingredients on the packages if you're not sure. Most packaged cookies and crackers contain hydrogenated oil and wheat. Definitely put them in the bag. Take the bag to your trash can and throw it out.

This may seem extreme, but it is time for you to take stock of how you are eating and, as a result, what is happening to your body. You need to eat foods that will nourish you and assist your body in healing. Your body needs all the help it can get and what you feed it is of utmost importance. It is your life that you are looking at here, not someone else's. You can do this!

I have told you what not to eat, now let's look at a list of what you need to eat:

1. Organic greens-spinach, broccoli, kale, radicchio, romaine, and any other greens you like. All greens in all their varieties. Choose the ones you like and then start adding different ones. Avoid eating the same thing every day.
2. Organic orange and red-colored vegetables- bell peppers, beets, and any other colorful vegetables you like. Try to eat what is in season. It will be less expensive and will provide you with the harmony of eating the way nature is intending through the farming cycle.
3. Organic fruits of all colors and flavors-fruits for snacks in mid-mornings and mid-afternoons will nourish and pamper you throughout the day. If you choose fruits of the season they will be sweet and will replace any craving you might have for a sweet snack.
4. Celtic salt or himalayan salt-these types of salts have minerals your body needs and have been minimally processed, unlike the processed salts. The processed salts do not have any nutritional value and are actually harmful to your body.

5. Organic meats-chicken, pork, red meat, and wild fish. If you eat meat make sure it is organic as much as possible. Grass-fed is also preferable. Although more expensive, you will find that you will eat less because it is much more dense and satisfying. So really, it will cost you the same, if not less. Eat only wild fish and never farmed fish.
6. Organic ghee-ghee is clarified butter and is believed to be very healing. It may be used to cook in high heat. Ghee also has medicinal healing properties aiding in your digestion. Our immune systems are directly tied to our digestion. Do not underestimate the importance of good digestion.
7. Organic butter, NOT margarine.
8. Organic cold pressed olive oil. Organic cold pressed coconut oil. It is not recommended to cook with olive oil as it begins to break down in high temperature. Use it in salads and even when baking, but not for frying. On the other hand, you can use coconut oil to cook. It is important that you eat oils. They are important for healthy brain function.
9. Organic avocados, nuts and seeds. The oils in these are essential. Pumpkin seeds are considered to be exceptionally good for MS and the nervous system. Eat a wide variety of seeds and nuts. They each have their own characteristics and healing nutrients.
10. Green tea, organic if possible. You may have it as iced tea or hot tea. I always have a pitcher of green tea in my refrigerator. There are varieties sold which have fruit essence in them and are tasty enough to not have to add sugar. Try different varieties until you find one you like. There is no reason for you to drink something you don't like.
11. Water. Plenty of filtered water. Make sure you stay hydrated throughout the day. It is very important to support your body's natural flow without stress of insufficient hydration. If you aren't doing it now, increase your water intake.
12. Organic beans, whichever you like. They are a great source of protein, especially if you are vegetarian or vegan. Try to have a variety of beans and in that way you are nourishing your body with a wide variety of necessary minerals and vitamins.

13. If you need to use sugar, only use raw organic sugar. Raw organic sugar is the only sugar that is alkaline. Try to keep the consumption of sugar to a minimum.
14. You may be wondering about coffee. I don't see anything wrong with having coffee. Try to have organic coffee. Try to drink it in moderation.

I think you get the idea. Organic is best when you can find it. You will avoid food that is genetically modified and contains pesticides if you eat organic. It may cost a little more, but what you'll find is that it is more satisfying and rich, and as a result you won't eat as much. Try to eat fresh whenever possible. In that way you won't have any unwanted additives or chemicals in your meals. Do not avoid oils. If you eat the right kinds of oils/fats, your body will be rejuvenated. Your brain needs the oils and fats.

Most importantly, observe how you feel. If you find that a certain food doesn't sit well with you, then avoid it. Even though it may be highly nutritious, it may be that you have a sensitivity to it. It's important that you be aware of food's effect on your body. I suggest you keep a journal of what you eat during the day and how you feel throughout the day. I believe that allergies and negative reactions to foods we eat contribute to MS and other autoimmune disorders. Listen closely to your body. Only you can know what or how something affects you. It's time to really start paying attention.

In addition:

1. Start your mornings with a warm cup of 1/2 lemon and water. This will make your body alkaline and set the tone for the day. Supporting alkalinity in the body is very important.
2. Take a half-teaspoon of organic turmeric and one teaspoon of raw honey and mix them together. The turmeric is an amazing anti inflammatory, along with other incredible properties and the honey is also very healing and has anti bacterial properties. You may want to take this at night before you go to bed. If you find that that is inconvenient, then take it any time you like. The point is for you to take it. Please don't take this lightly. It is very, very

beneficial for you in so many ways. If you find it is not pleasant, add warm water and lemon to it and make a tea out of it.

3. Take vitamin D-3 every day.
4. If you are on medication, take milk thistle. The medicines are very hard on the liver. Milk thistle helps the liver to process and eliminate the chemicals and stay healthy.
5. Take a fish oil capsule daily. This is recommended for better brain function.
6. Take a vitamin B complex. This supports a healthy nervous system. If you are vegetarian, chances are you aren't getting enough vitamin B-12 or the others as well, and is essential that you have them.

Once you begin implementing the changes to your diet and incorporating the supplements, you will notice a change within a month. You will find yourself feeling lighter and stronger. Your digestion will become regular. Your skin and your hair will begin to feel healthier. And this is the first step to loving yourself and being compassionate with your body.

At the time of eating, take time to eat. Before starting to eat, be aware that you are very, very lucky to have food on your plate. Be grateful for that. Then eat in as serene an environment as possible. Take the opportunity to taste and experience your food. The gift of your food. Try not to ever eat in anger. Take meal time as an important part of the day for you and for your family to enjoy and share. This will give the food you eat the ability to act as a nourishing and healing agent. Always, always bring the awareness to how grateful you are for the food you are able to have. Gratitude is the state that brings change to your life in a positive way. Gratitude is what will change your life...

Exercise

Without question, you have to exercise. I am a big proponent of walking. In walking you are doing a weight bearing form of exercise which is essential for not only your muscles, but also your bones. The movement of a brisk walk also gets the digestive juices flowing and helps with better digestion.

Mentally, a walk will awaken the neurons in the brain and will keep you alert. New neurons will begin to grow with every step and clarity will come as a result. Try to walk outdoors where you are in contact with nature. At some point take off your shoes and feel the grass under your feet. Ground yourself and connect with the earth below you and nature around you. Be aware, with gratitude, of the world around you. Try to walk for 30 minutes or more. After exercising spend a few minutes practicing mental exercises. A crossword puzzle, Sudoku, learn a language, or practice an instrument. Anything that will stimulate your brain. This is essential to help new neurons continue to grow after physically exercising. Here's the science behind this theory: New neurons begin to grow when we exercise physically. Once we stop our physical exercise, what happens to the new neurons? Well, if we then focus on our minds and exercise our minds, those new neurons will live. If we don't exercise our minds those new neurons will not continue to grow, but instead will shrink as if they had never been there in the first place. In learning this, I hope you will understand the importance of following physical exercise with mental exercise. We can regenerate our brains. We can help our brains become strong and healthy. Let there be no doubt about that.

If you are not able to walk very far at this point, don't worry. Begin by walking for five minutes and start adding a little more every few days. Your muscles will benefit and begin to get stronger. You will slowly start building up stamina. This will be especially true when you start implementing all the other tools in this book.

If you are not able to walk at all at this point, don't worry. Sit with your eyes closed and feel yourself walking from wherever you are sitting to a point close by. Do this for a few minutes every day; once or twice a day or more if you would like. If you practice mentally feeling yourself walking, your muscles will benefit and begin to get stronger. Your body responds to your mind. There are studies in which people who mentally exercise without movement have muscle build up as if they had physically done it. Be aware that your body doesn't really know the difference, if you put mental effort in combination with the feeling of performing the exercises. When I say feeling, I mean *feeling.* Even though physically you can't do it, let the muscles express themselves as if they are. You will be surprised by the muscle build up that will occur. Once you start implementing every tool you're given in this book, you will start getting stronger. Don't forget to exercise the brain immediately after, no matter what your situation is. Once you become strong enough to start walking, take it easy and do a little at a time and progressively add more as in the instructions above.

Stress management

In my experience, managing your stress is *the* single most important part of this process. It's time you become very aware of the effect of what you do has on you. Stress in itself is not what has the negative effect. It is necessary to have stress in given situations. It is the perception of stress that is what does the damage. If you spend much of your time worrying about something that happened in the past… If you spend much of your time worrying about things that may happen in the future, which will probably never happen, you are spending your life in worry and stress. This constant level of stress is very hard on the body and eventually the body gets sick. Your body cannot take being in fight or flight mode 24 hours a day. Physiologically it's a very damaging process that creates autoimmune responses in the body. It's time to change that right now. Not tomorrow, not next week, but now.

Begin this process by taking the word "should" out of your vocabulary. Instead, replace it with the words "need to," "have to," "want to." If you cannot use those words in doing something, then chances are that you don't really need to do it. Not only do you not need to do it, but you don't have any desire to do it. In that case, DON'T DO IT. I'm not telling to check out in your life, on the contrary, I am asking you to do the things that give you joy. Take stock of the obligations that you have today. How many of them are optional? How many of them deep down bring you joy? Not because you are expected to do it, but because they truly bring you joy. If they don't, then it's time to step aside and let someone else take over, who will find joy in it. In the same way you cleaned out your food pantry, it's now time to do the same with your life.

Do the things that you need to do, like work, take care of your loved ones, and so on. Do these things from a place of love. Be aware of how lucky you are to have a job and loved ones. Volunteer for only those things you love, and say *no* to any others you don't want to do because it's OK to say *no*. Continue to stay involved in your life, your children's lives, your family's life with joy that they are a part of your life. Be grateful for all you have. Whatever you do, do *not* use MS as an excuse not to do something. It will not leave you if you use it as an excuse. If you can't because you're tired, then say that you are tired, not that you are sick. Start seeing yourself as a healthy person with an off day. We all have off days and I want you to start thinking in those terms. Be compassionate with yourself. Start your day by loving yourself. Drink your lemon water. Be aware you are doing this to help your body become healthy. Love the perfectly imperfect being you are. Spread that love every chance you get. Release the fear. All fear. Be aware that most of your fears are self-created. Take comfort in knowing this and shift to a place of love instead.

Spend time with those you want to spend time with. Spend time with those who are loving and kind to you. Their love will help you. Take the time to love them back. You can do so by expressing that love or by doing things which you know would make their lives better. In giving lies the receiving. Be very aware of that. Know that as important as it is for you to focus on yourself, it's just as important to share love with others who may need it. Stay away from negative people with negative emotions. If you watch movies or television shows, watch those which are inspiring, rewarding, lighthearted, funny or happy and bring your spirits up. Those emotions are healing emotions. Let them start to work. There are many studies of emotions on physiology supporting what I'm recommending. If you incorporate all of the suggestions above you will see the difference within a very short period of time. Become aware of the small shifts in your mind and body. As the shifts grow, always remember to be grateful. Live in gratitude and watch your world become a place of grace.

CHAPTER 13

What Is Yoga?

Now let me explain further how to bring your body and mind to a place of balance and health. I know firsthand that reading lengthy books or directions is sometimes difficult for people who have MS, so I've tried making each chapter as brief as possible. Don't worry, I will try to be brief here too, but will get the information to you as thoroughly as possible.

So, let's start from the beginning.

What is yoga? The best description I have heard that resonated with me as a Westerner is: "Yoga is the science of the union of mind and body."

What does that mean?

I want you to be very clear on what yoga is. In order to apply what you will be learning you have to understand what it is.

Let's break it down:

A *science*—that means it is not a religion. Yoga is not composed of religious beliefs. No matter what your religion is, you can practice yoga without it interfering with your religious beliefs.

Union—the joining and becoming one.

Mind—the thoughts and therefore the "states of mind" and feelings.

Body—the physical, arms, legs, and so on.

So our goal is to unite body with the mind. A mind that is relaxed and balanced, free of judgment and ready to pass that balance along to the body, as they are one.

What we think has an effect on our bodies. If your mind is filled with negative, fearful thoughts, your body will become stressed. Stress will breed *dis-ease.* If on the other hand you can replace negative thoughts with relaxing, balanced thoughts, your body will be balanced as well.

Stress is the result of our perception of a situation. What to one person can be an adventure, to another can be a dangerous situation. What to one person is a challenge, to another is a problem. Are you following this? It's not the stress that creates problems; it's our perception of a situation through the lens of fear. I'm not saying that there are no problems, or that they are not real. What I am saying is that we can resolve them without stressing our minds and bodies. When we come to a bump in the road, we drive over it. It may slow us down, but that's okay. We have learned that our bodies and minds are two separate entities, involved in separate processes. But, if you take a moment and really give it some thought, it won't take you long to realize how ridiculous a notion this is. Unless the mind sends the right signals, we can't move our legs. If the mind doesn't coordinate properly, our vision, speech, and other body parts will not function properly. Yes, this is done without any apparent thought process, but it is in fact the mind which does it.

In learning yoga:

You learn the way in which your mind and body are intertwined and connected. In order to have a healthy body you must have a healthy mind.

You learn the effect of breath on the body. You learn how to channel that breath into healing energy.

You learn the power of your thoughts, but you also learn the importance of giving your mind a break.

You learn that the space between the thoughts is more important than the thoughts themselves in your journey to healing.

Your learning process will be split up into parts, every part being just as important as the other. Neglecting one would have an impact on the success of the others. You will learn postures/asanas, pranayama/breathing techniques and meditation. Each plays a very important role.

Your ability level is what will determine your progress. It is important that you always keep in mind everyone's body is different. There is no room for comparison. You do what your body and mind allow and you will progress with practice. Within that frame also keep in mind that some days are better than others and that's okay, just do your best. There is no room for stress or fretting over your progress. Diligently practice every day and progress will be made in the way it needs to happen. Let go and let it happen… Enjoy…

Asanas – Postures

Let me take a minute to address the common perception of asanas.

For many people who have never practiced yoga, the mental picture that comes to mind is often of someone in an incredibly difficult posture, if not standing on their head, or into a pretzel, pretty close to it. I am here to tell you that couldn't be further from the truth. Yes, there are those who can do some very difficult postures and feel very relaxed, but in order to benefit from yoga that's not necessary. On the contrary, I think you will be surprised by the effect that very subtle movements can have on your body as well as your mind.

The asanas are a series of physical postures to help your body get stronger, more limber, relaxed and for you to be able to sit in meditation without any stress. You will find certain parts of your body will have more stiffness than others. Some asanas will be more difficult than others as a result. That's perfectly normal. In fact the less you are able to do an asana the more you should do it. Stiffness in any part of the body should be avoided. Toxins rest in those stiff parts because we tend to not move those parts. That's the reason they have become stiff in the first place. As you practice, remember to always back out immediately of anything causing you pain. I'm not telling you not to push yourself into a posture and relax in it, but definitely do it without pain. You are asked to do those that are at your ability level, and to truly listen to your body. As you progress, you will add more. With the repetition of asanas on a daily basis you will be rerouting your brain and forming new paths for information. Within these new paths will come progress. You may feel the results right away or it may take a while, but just know that you are training your brain and that will help with cognitive, physical, visual and other symptoms you might be experiencing. Your body will start to become balanced, and as that happens you will start to feel vitality and health coming back. It will be an adventure into a beautiful progression into wellness.

Breathing Techniques

It is extremely important that you learn to breathe correctly. Initially I want you to focus on just breathing correctly. Once you are comfortable with that, then you move on to other types of breaths to benefit your body in different ways. I will give you an exact road map to this with step by step directions. The effect of this on your mind and body is truly amazing. I CAN'T EMPHASIZE ENOUGH THE IMPORTANCE OF BREATH. Breath is what keeps us alive, and nourishes us. Without it, we can't function. Without proper breathing we don't nourish our bodies properly, hence inviting problems.

Relaxation through breathing is key; relaxation of the body as well as the mind. One cannot be relaxed without the other being relaxed. In order for your body to heal, it needs to have total relaxation time, to give it the chance to heal. Unless the mind is relaxed, there will be tension in some part of the body. Ultimate relaxation of both is what will take place.

Meditations

A stressed mind is a tired mind. A stressed mind has a difficult time absorbing and learning. A stressed mind passes the stress to the body and that is where the body may feel pain or get sick. Just as your body needs rest, so does the mind. Even when we are sleeping, our minds are busy dreaming and solving our days' situations. However, if you give the mind a break from thought all together throughout your day, you will find benefits that are all encompassing to your mind and body.

This brings us to the all-important part of yoga: meditation. Meditation addresses all these issues. You will be handed a road map to help you achieve a good meditation practice. Again, progressing as you practice. There is no room for comparison. Just know that your practice is yours alone, and your own experience. Honor that. Your experience may be completely different from someone else's, but that doesn't make one better than the other. Some days will be better than others. That's okay, it's all part of the experience. I assure you that you will be very pleasantly surprised by the results. Possibly ecstatic! I know I am.

All asanas, breathing practices and meditations will be split into levels. Depending on your physical abilities, you may progress faster in your breathing and meditation levels. That is ABSOLUTELY PERFECT. The progression of your breathing and meditation are what will aid in your physical recovery and if you have cognitive issues, your cognitive recovery as well.

One final note before we begin:

I want you to be aware of the things that make you feel good. I want you to be aware of those that don't. I am talking about music, books, television, movies, people, and anything else. There is no room for negativity from here on out. If that means not watching the news, don't watch the news. If that means saying *no* to people, please say *no.* Do not feel guilty. You are now in a state of recovery, healing and living. *Do* the things you *want* to do, not the things you *should* do. *Do* the things you have to do with gratitude, that you can do them at all. It means a shift in attitude. It means you have a whole new attitude toward life and the adventures coming your way. Be kind and loving to others, but most importantly, be kind to yourself. That includes surrounding yourself with people and an environment which support your shift to joy and hope.

It's time to lose your fears. Fear is a paralyzing emotion. Fear is a negative emotion. Fear takes a very heavy toll on your body. I won't go into the medical aspects of it; you can research it if you are curious. Just know that it is very important for your well being to drop your fear. Fear of what might happen if… What might happen when… What has happened in the past and your guilt about it… There is no room for that anymore. What will happen, will happen, what has happened has happened, and no amount of worrying will help. *But*, if you take life and run with it and try to give it your all, you will be *living. Believe* you can get better, and then you can leave the fears behind. Let joy fill your heart and every cell in your body. Find new adventures that fit your circumstances right now.

Have you always wanted to paint? Then do it. You think you don't have talent? How do you know? Try it! What do you have to lose? You might be pleasantly surprised at how much fun putting paint on paper or canvass can be. How about if you try learning to play the piano or the guitar, or maybe learning another language. The point is, try new things to stimulate your body, your brain and your spirit. The key is to start using parts of your brain you have never used. Lift your spirit in ways you have never lifted it. Love yourself and others in a way you have never loved before.

Now let's begin the journey to recovery together. I will be with you every step of the way.

CHAPTER 14

Asanas / Postures

We will be covering a set of postures that make up the best-known sequence in Hatha yoga—the Sun Salutation or Surya Namaskar. Each posture covers a different part of the body. Even if you already practice yoga and know that you know how to do this, please approach the process in the way I'm requesting. Before you attempt to practice the Sun Salutation, I would like you to take one of the twelve postures per day in the order presented. Repeat it 11 times in the morning and 11 times in the evening before bed. If you feel that you need more than one day to understand the posture, then spend two or three or more days on it. The point is for you to be comfortable with the posture and then incorporate the breathing, and then feel the flow of the breath throughout the body. Try to relax in the posture for a few breaths and enjoy how it settles into you and the effect it has on your body. As you progress, practice each individually. Adding each one as you go, but do not bring them together until you have practiced each one individually and understand and are comfortable with it. So, for example, if you are comfortable with the first posture after a day or two, then begin to practice the second one. So that day you will be practicing the first one and then the second one individually. Once the second one is understood add the third one the next day. Then you will be doing the first, second and third one that day. But do them individually, not in flow sequence together just yet. Continue doing this with all of the postures until you are very comfortable with each one. What I mean by comfortable, is that you feel the effect that posture has on your body, because you have taken the time to observe it and relax in it. Once you feel comfortable with each posture, you can put them all together in sequence and perform the Sun Salutation/Surya Namaskar. Take the sequence in a slow, mindful manner. Be very aware of your body and breath with every movement. After having comfortably practiced the sun salutation you can then add the triangle pose or Trikonasana to your practice. This pose will be very beneficial for you and will make you feel strong and light at the same time.

After your practice each day, no matter what you have practiced, whether it's one asana/posture 11 times or a full sun salutation, finish the asanas by lying in Savasana. In Savasana you lie on your back with your feet twelve to eighteen inches apart. Your arms are extended at your sides on the ground. Your palms need to be about six inches away from your body and will be facing up. Stay there for at least two minutes and allow the effect of your postures to settle into your body in total relaxation. Then very gently turn onto your right side and use your arms and hands to sit up slowly. You will find detailed instructions and pictures in the following pages. Above all enjoy your practice. It is meant to bring you relaxation and healing.

Surya Namaskar – Sun Salutation

Surya Namaskar covers every part of your body. From the crown of your head to the tips of your toes you will engage your whole body. It is a flow of 12 postures/asanas that will strengthen, energize and relax you at a physical as well as mental level. I suggest you take each asana individually and get to know it very well. Get to know how your body feels as you are moving through the posture and also as you settle yourself in the posture releasing any tension and relaxing. It is a very intimate and personal relationship you will develop in this process. It is the process of getting to know your body and how it works. It is the process of discovering where you have stiffness and how to release that stiffness. It is the process of discovering how to be in the moment, in the *now* as you feel your body and breath flow in harmony and support. Each asana addresses a different part of the body, but be aware that when you are putting them all together you are creating a magnificent dance in which your awareness and release of judgment are important. Begin by performing each posture to the best of your ability.

Alignment is important, but remember not all bodies are built the same, so listen to yours. If you find your body aligns just slightly differently than expected, honor it and know that this is where you need to be. Always move into a posture slowly and gently, without any jerking and without any pain. If at any time you feel pain, immediately, but slowly back out and gently place yourself in that posture in a way where you are not in any pain. A little pressure or discomfort is okay, but pain is definitely not. Listen to your body. Be aware of your breath. Your progression in each of the postures will flow in the way and when it needs to happen. There is no goal in this process, only a journey. In performing any of the asanas, always give yourself a few moments before you begin. Begin with your feet parallel and approximately hip width apart—enough for you to be stable. Find yourself physically centered. By this, I mean, let the weight of your body be centered and evenly distributed on your feet. As you are breathing in lift your shoulders up and back and as you breathe out let them relax slowly down. You are standing straight, but relaxed. Your arms are hanging free and loose at your sides. Close your eyes and breathe in through your nose and out through the center of your lips. Slowly and gently, let your breath bring you to this present moment. Take as long as you need. There is no rush. If you cannot stand, follow the process sitting down. Now, slowly bring your palms together. Your thumbs are at the base of your throat and your chin is cradled between your index fingers and middle fingers. Again, stay here for a moment and be with your breath. When you are ready you can begin taking the following steps below.

Initially, don't worry about the breath. Just try to do the postures and understand them. Then incorporate the breath as instructed and you will feel the beauty of the support of the breath. You will feel what it is to be in harmony. Each asana is numbered below. Do them in the sequence in which they are numbered. Enjoy the process. Now, with your palms together, thumbs at your voice box and index finger and middle finger cradling your chin, slide them down your chest, without letting them separate at the base, until the thumbs are in the middle of your chest roughly at your heart level, as you're breathing out. Let's begin.

Surya Namaskar/Sun Salutation

1. Pranamasana - Your palms are together in prayer pose, while standing with feet parallel. With the thumbs pressed against your chest, feel your heart beating. Become aware of the life force within you. Breathe. You can remain here for as many breaths as you'd like.

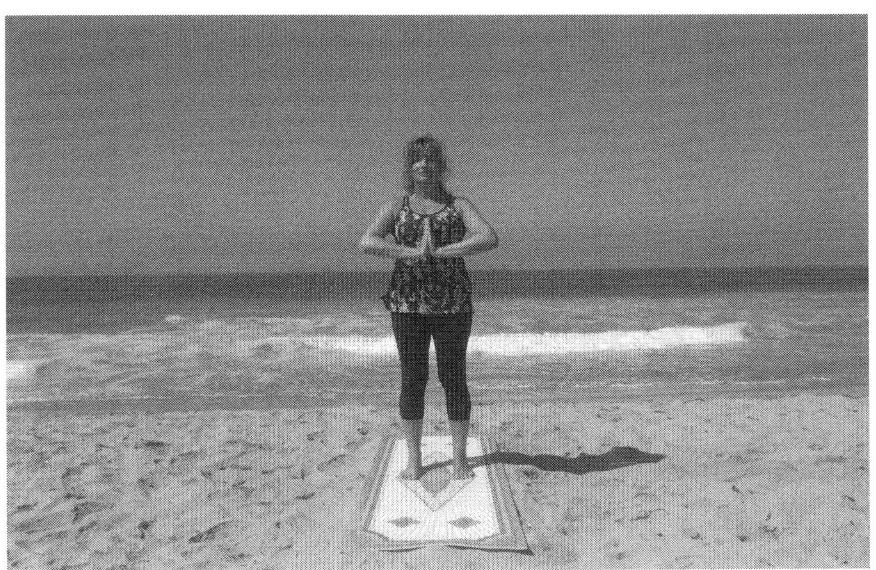

2. Hasta Utthanasana - Raise your arms, palms together- as you are breathing in. Keeping your eyes open tilt your head back and bend back slightly; enough to feel it at your sternum as you are breathing in. Slowly bring your head up straight with your arms overhead and palms together and finish that breath in. If you decide to stay in the bent position longer you can breathe in and out, but make sure as you're coming up you are breathing in and your eyes are open at all times.

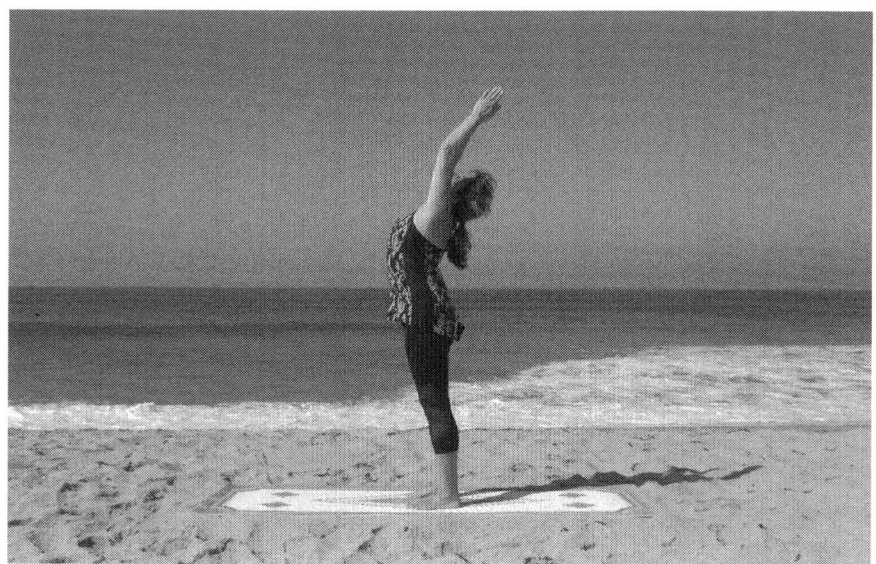

3. Padahastasana - arms straight overhead, palms together, coming forward folding from the waist taking the head toward the knees, hands to the feet, legs or holding ankle from the back or as close to that as possible. As you come forward you are breathing out. Remember that in order to bend forward you have to have an empty chest and belly, so you breathe out as you are doing it. To come out of it go up in the same way you came down.

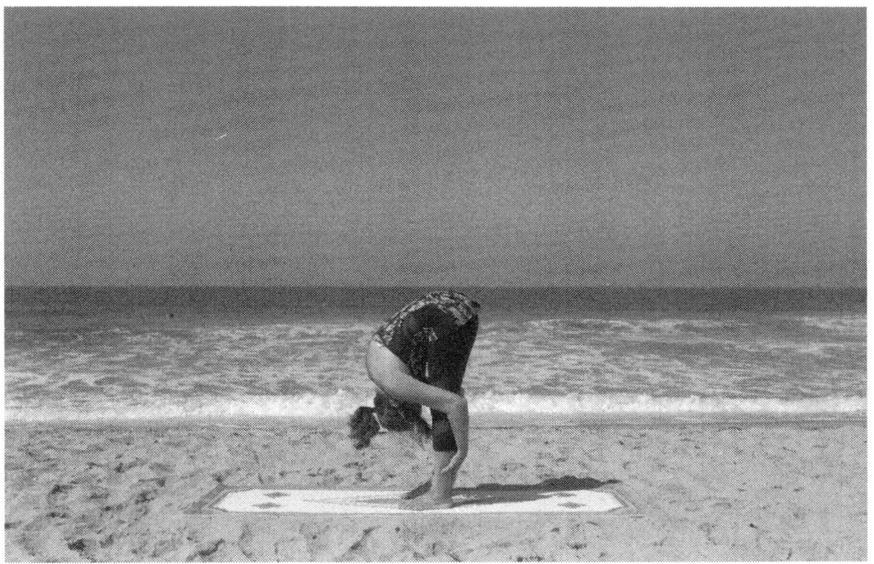

4. Ashwa Sanchalanasana - Take the left leg back, with the left knee and top of the left foot on the ground, right knee bent, back is arched, head up and back, hands are on either side of the right foot, fingers in line with the toes. Right knee is over the right ankle. Try to bring your hips forward and down as close to the ground as you can. Breathe in going into the posture. Remain here, breathe and relax.

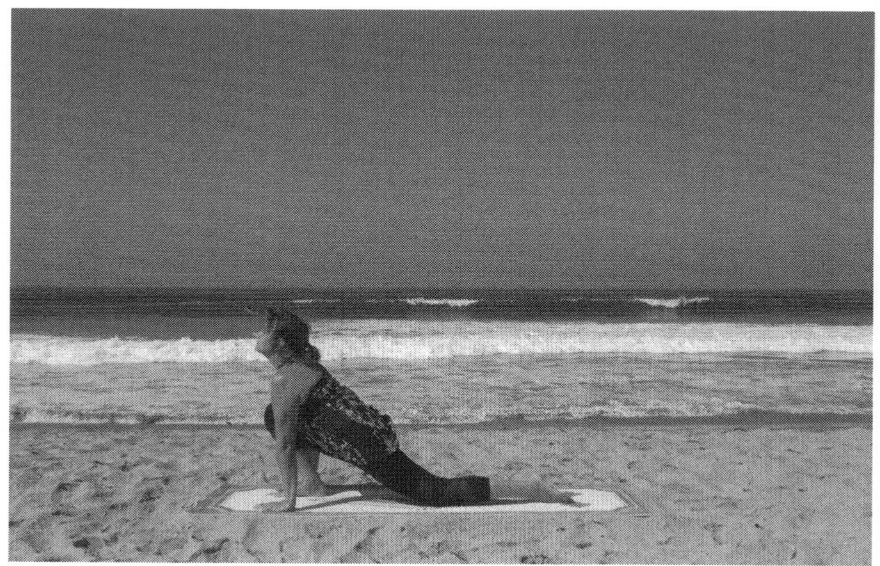

5. Parvatasana – You are on your hands and knees. The right foot is in line with the left foot, the knees are on the ground hip width apart. Lift the knees off the ground, go on to your toes, push your hips up as high as you can and then take the heels down as close to touching the ground as possible. Your legs are straight, and there is no bend at the knees, if possible. The chin tucks in to the chest and your arms are straight. Do not overstretch your heals. Honor what your body can do. Breathe out as you go into this posture.

Breathe gently while in the posture, it will not be a full breath because your chin is at your chest.

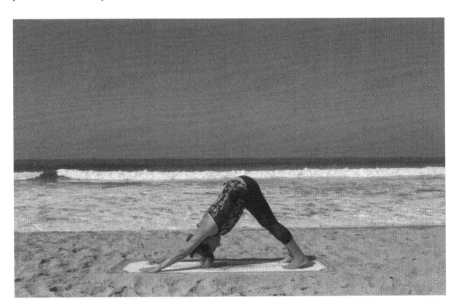

6. Ashtanga Namaskara – The hands and knees are on the ground. Bring the chest in line with the hands and lower the chest onto the ground, your chin goes on the ground. Your belly is off the ground. Toes are curled under, pointing toward your body. Breathe out as you are going into it. Your chin, chest, knees and toes are all on the ground. Feel the stretch in your throat and throughout your spine.

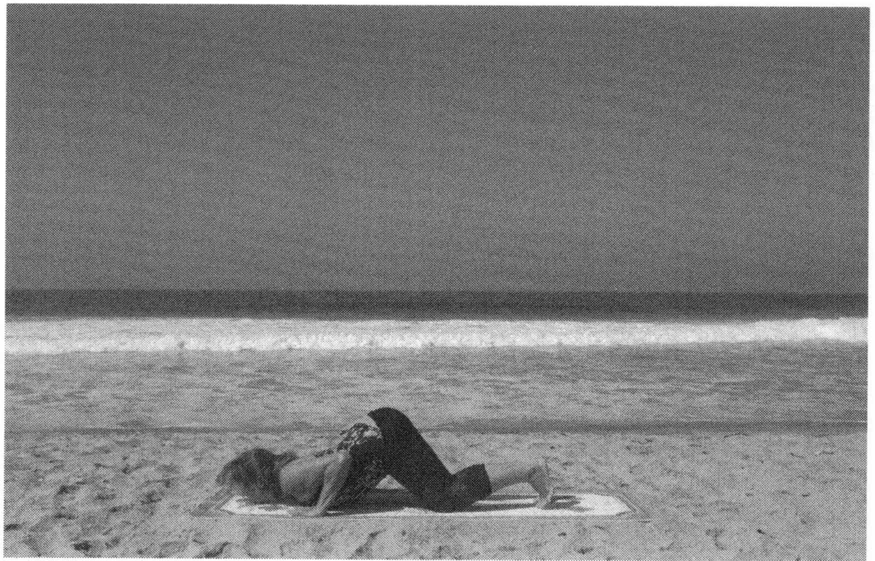

7. Bhujangasana – Lie on your stomach with your forehead touching the ground. Your arms are bent close to your body and your palms are under your shoulders. Slowly slide your head forward and up and leave your chin in contact with the ground stretching your neck. Breathe in as you do this and breathe out. Slowly raise your chest off the ground with your stomach still on the ground and stay there, breathe in as you do this and breathe out. Your stomach, hips, legs and tops of the feet are on the ground. Arms are close to the body- breathe in. Straighten the arms, your stomach is off the ground and continue to arch the back and your face is up and back. Your hips as close to the ground as possible but always honor what your body can do. Breathe fully in and out in this posture. To get out of the posture go through the steps in the reverse order. Lower your hips, lower your stomach, lower your chest, bring the chin to the ground, and finally bring the forehead to the ground.

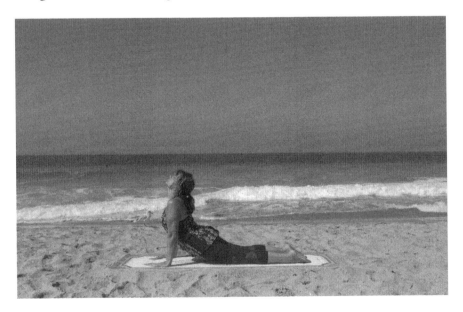

8. Parvatasana - You are on your hands and knees. The right foot is in line with the left foot, the knees are on the ground hip width apart. Lift the knees off the ground, go on to your toes, push your hips up as high as you can and then take the heels down as close to touching the ground as possible. Your legs are straight, and there is no bend at the knees, if possible. The chin tucks in to the chest and your arms are straight. Do not overstretch your heals. Honor what your body can do. Breathe out as you go into this posture. Breathe gently while in the posture, it will not be a full breath because your chin is at your chest.

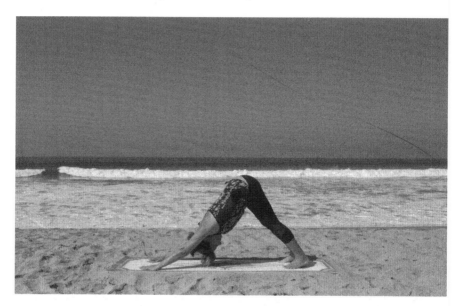

9. Ashwa Sanchalanasana – Take the right leg back, with the right knee and top of the right foot on the ground, left knee bent, back is arched, head up and back, hands are on either side of the left foot, fingers in line with the toes. The left knee is over the left ankle. Try to bring your hips forward and down as close to the ground as you can. Breathe in going into the posture. Remain here, breathe and relax.

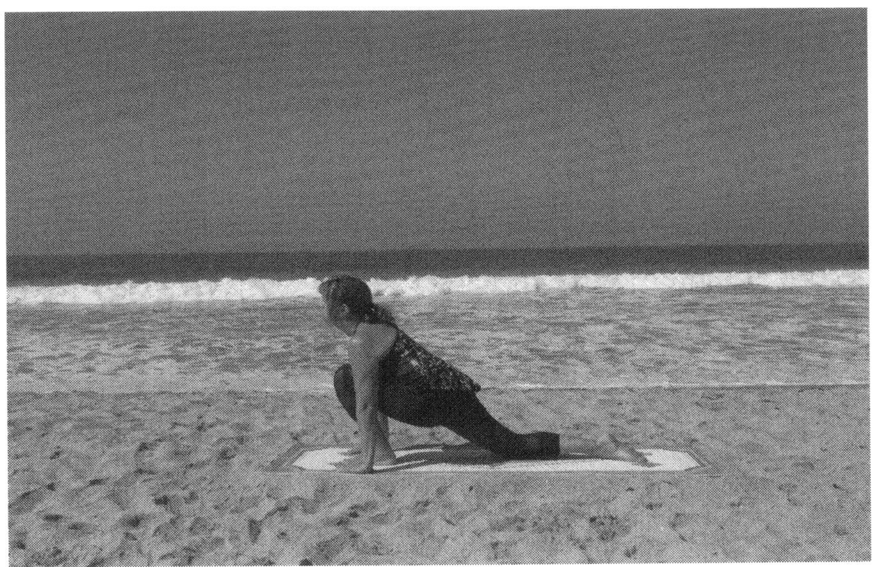

10. Padahastasana – Arms straight, palms together, coming forward folding from the waist taking the head toward the knees, hands to the feet, legs or holding your ankles from the back or as close to that as possible. As you come forward you are breathing out. Remember that in order to bend forward you have to have an empty chest and belly, so you breathe out as you are doing it.

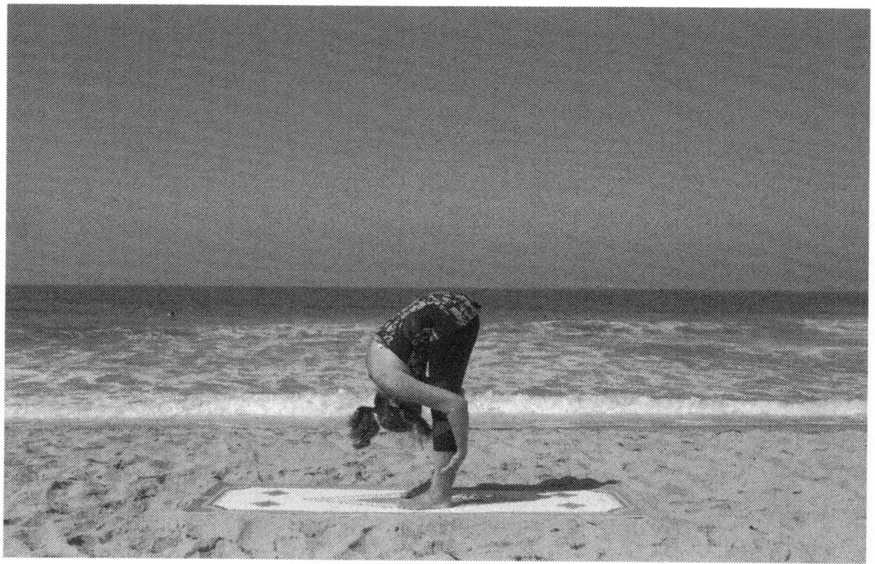

11. Hasta Utthanasana – Raise your arms straight overhead, palms together- as you are breathing in. Keeping your eyes open, tilt your head back and bend back slightly; enough to feel it at your sternum as you are breathing in. Slowly bring your head up straight with your arms overhead and palms together and finish that breath in. If you decide to stay in the bent position longer you can breathe in and out, but make sure as you're coming up you are breathing in and your eyes are open at all times.

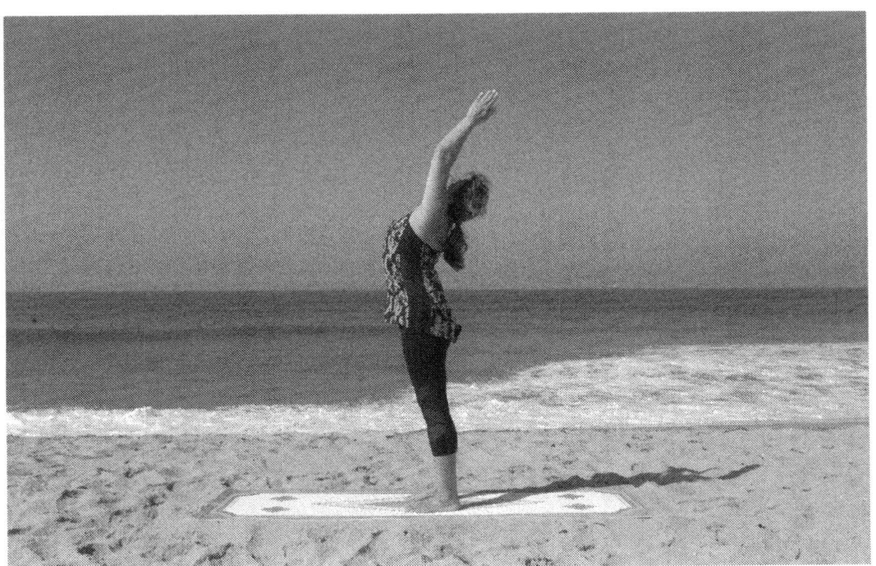

12. Pranamasana - Your palms are together in prayer pose, while standing with feet parallel. With the thumbs pressed against your chest, feel your heart beating. Become aware of the life force within you. Breathe. You can remain here for as many breaths as you'd like.

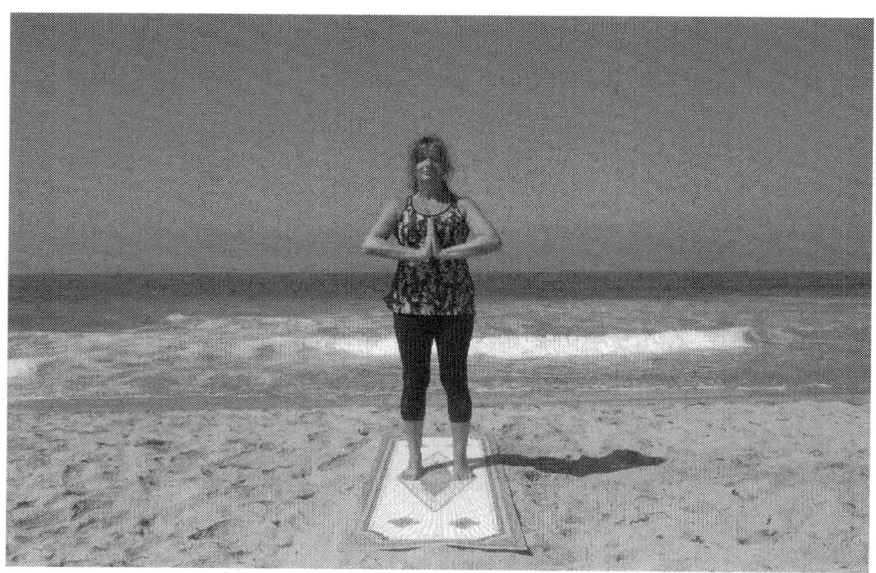

Go to transcendingms.com and we will perform Surya Namaskar together once you are ready to put all the postures together.

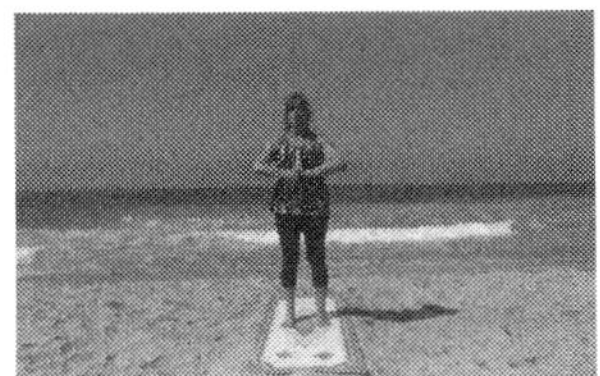

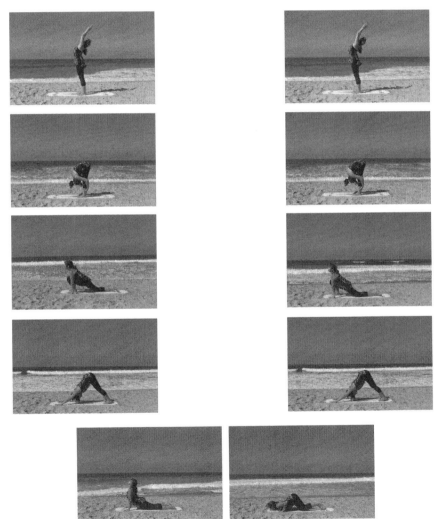

Modified Surya Namaskar/Sun Salutation

1. Pranamasana – While you are sitting. Your palms are together in prayer pose. With the thumbs pressed against your chest, feel your heart beating. Become aware of the life force within you. Breathe. You can remain here for as many breaths as you'd like. Then as you breathe out, straighten the arms and extend them at shoulder level with the palms together.

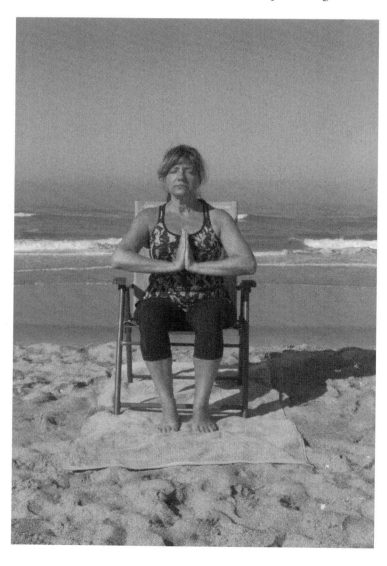

2. Hasta Utthanasana – While you are sitting. Raise your arms, palms together- as you are breathing in. Keeping your eyes open tilt your head back and bend back slightly; enough to feel it at your sternum as you are breathing in. Slowly bring your head up straight with your arms overhead and palms together and finish that breath in. If you decide to stay in the bent position longer you can breathe in and out, but make sure as you're coming up you are breathing in and your eyes are open at all times.

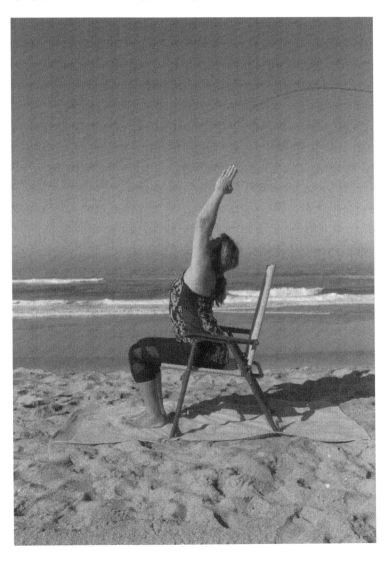

3. Padahastasana – While you are sitting. Your arms are straight up, palms are together. Breathing out come forward taking your head to your knees, hands to the feet or holding ankles from the back or as close to that as possible.

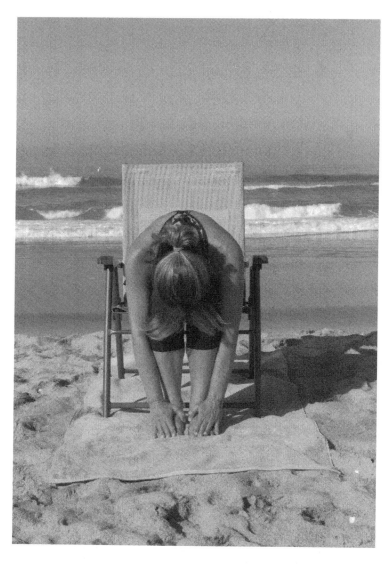

4. Ashwa Sanchalanasana – While you are sitting. Breathing in. Adjust the body up gently with a straight back. Raise the right knee toward the chest holding it with both hands, tilting your head back or keeping it straight if you cannot tilt it back.

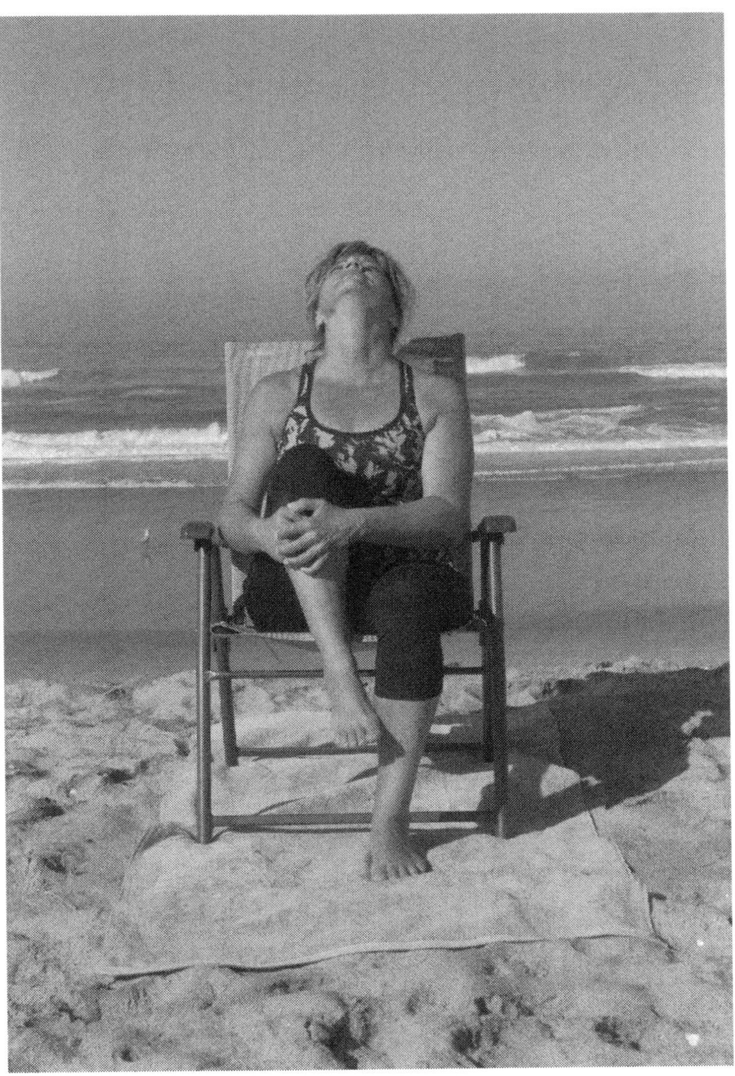

5. Parvatasana – While you are sitting. As you are breathing out. Bring your hands to your knees, elbows straight, touch your chin to your chest.

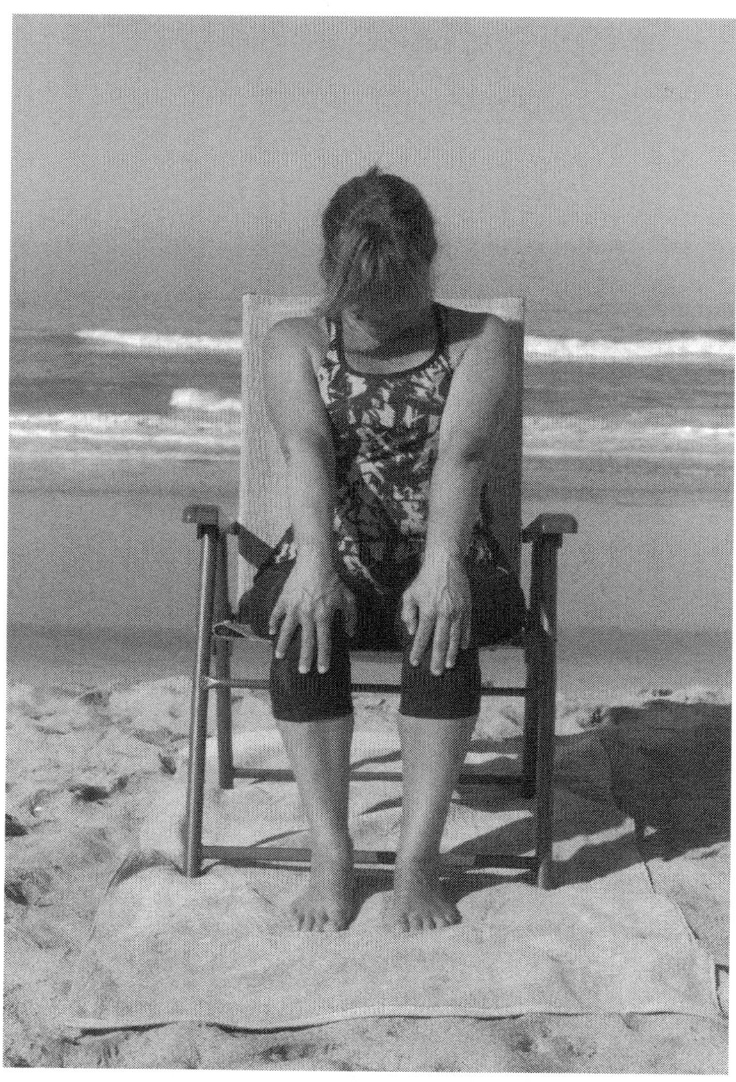

6. Ashtanga Namaskara – While you are sitting. Chest on the lap, hands on the knees, elbows outward, head in line with the back face beyond the knees, head as if looking straight ahead.

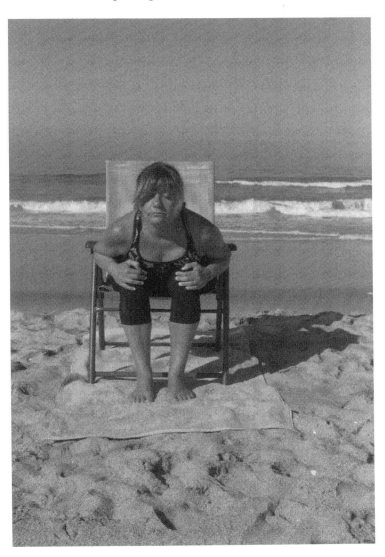

7. Bhujangasana – While you are sitting. Begin with your chest in your lap and hands on the knees. Lift chest off the lap half way by straightening your arms, arching the back and your face toward the sky. Breathe in as you go through the posture.

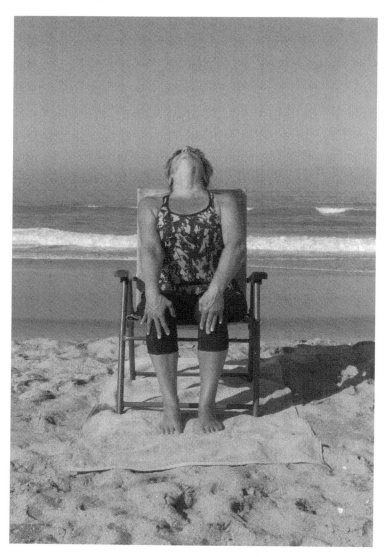

8. Parvatasana – While you are sitting. As you are breathing out. Bring your hands to your knees, elbows straight, touch your chin to your chest

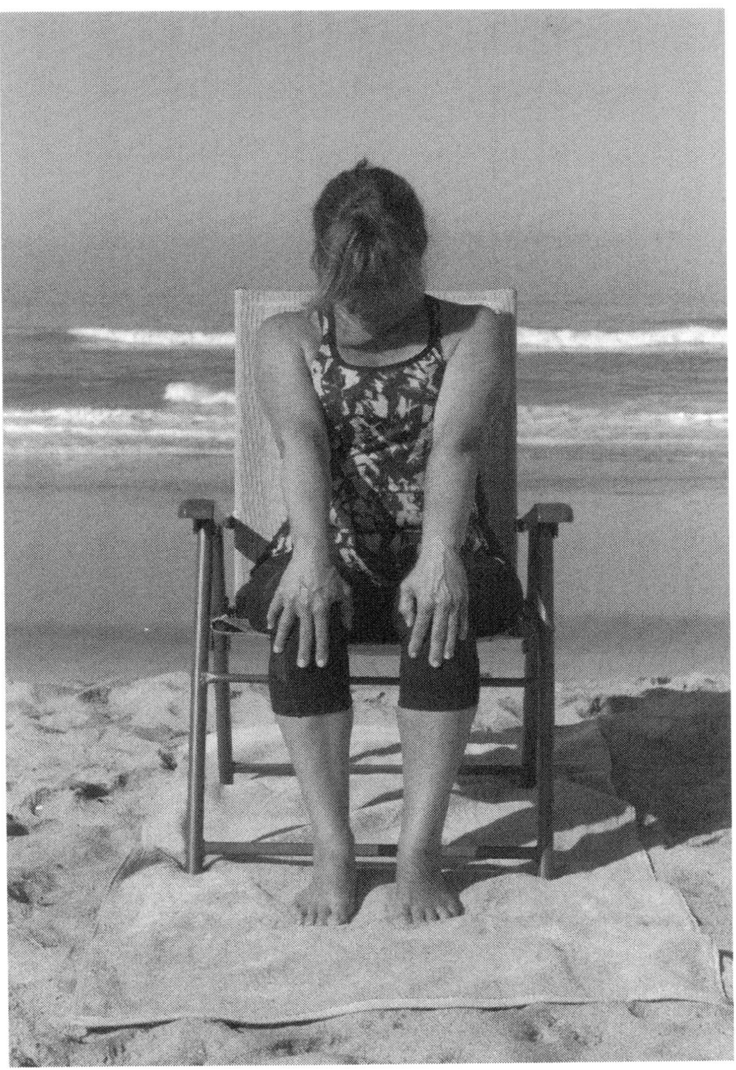

9. Ashwa Sanchalanasana – While you are sitting. Breathing in- Adjust the body up gently with a straight back. Raise the left knee toward the chest holding it with both hands, tilting your head back or keeping it straight if you cannot tilt it back..

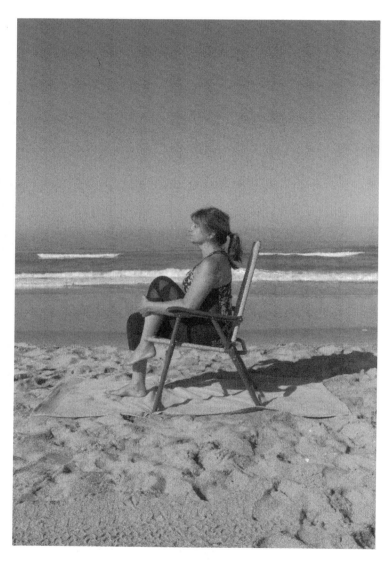

10. Padahastasana – While you are sitting. Your arms are straight above your head and your palms are together. Breathing out - come forward taking your head to your knees, hands to the feet or holding ankles from the back or as close to that as possible.

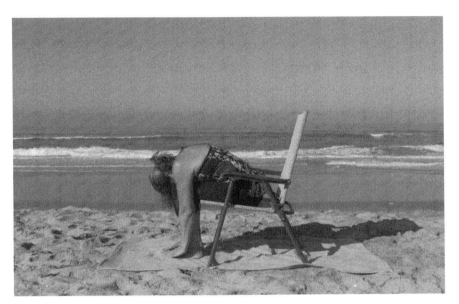

11. Hasta Utthanasana – While you are sitting. Raise your arms, palms together- as you are breathing in. Keeping your eyes open tilt your head back and bend back slightly; enough to feel it at your sternum as you are breathing in. Slowly bring your head up straight with your arms overhead and palms together and finish that breath in. If you decide to stay in the bent position longer you can breathe in and out, but make sure as you're coming up you are breathing in and your eyes are open at all times.

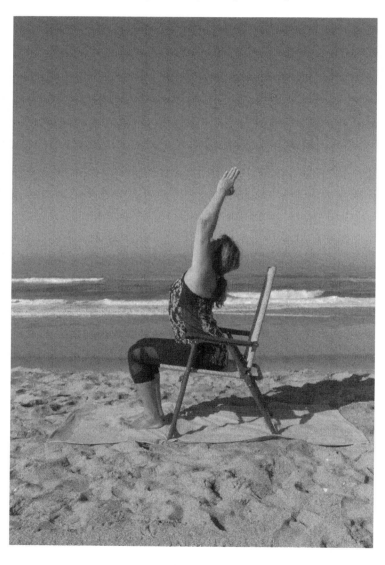

12. Pranamasana – While you are sitting. Your palms are together in prayer pose. With the thumbs pressed against your chest, feel your heart beating. Become aware of the life force within you. Breathe. You can remain here for as many breaths as you'd like. Then as you breathe out release you hands slowly and gently.

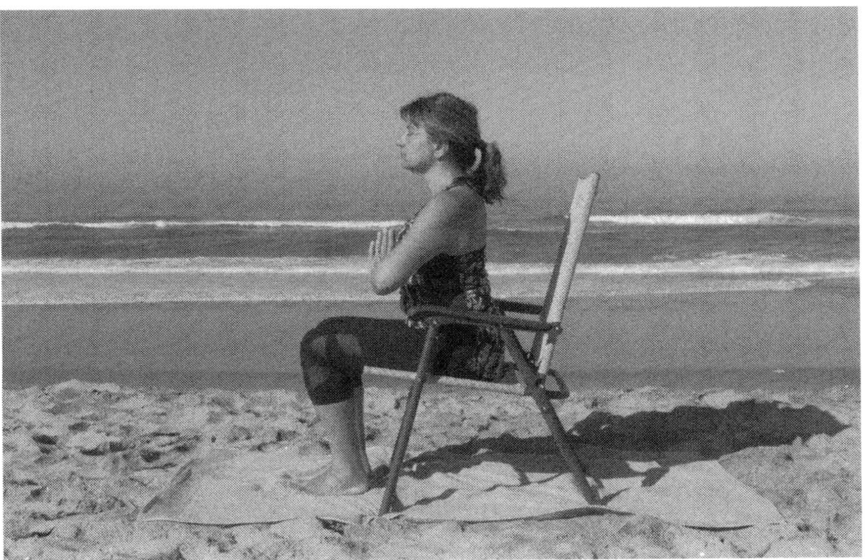

Go to transcendingms.com and we will perform Modified Surya Namaskar together once you are ready to put all the postures together.

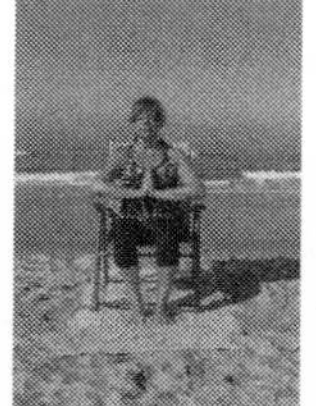
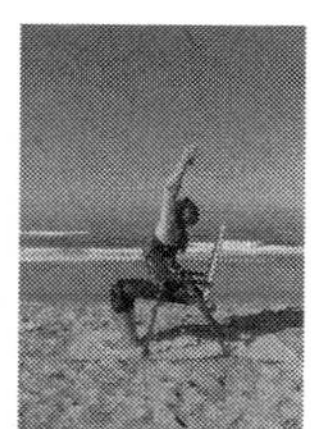
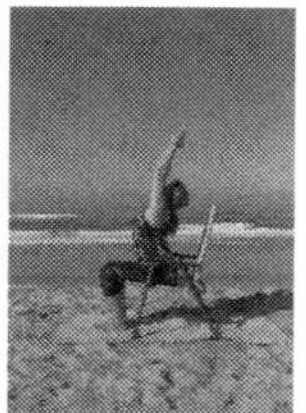
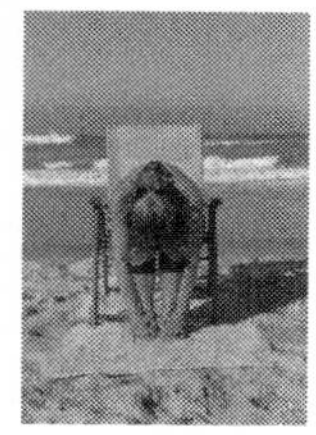
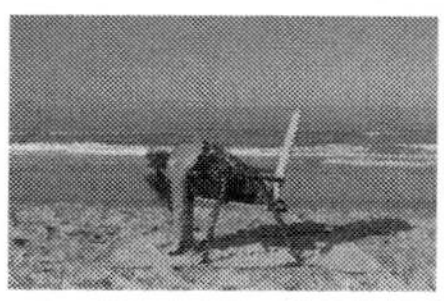
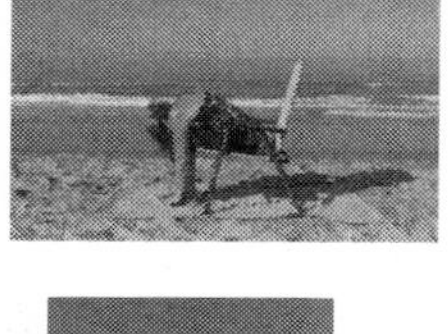
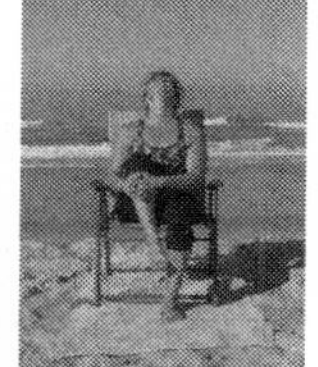
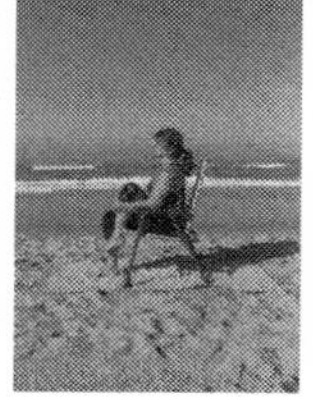
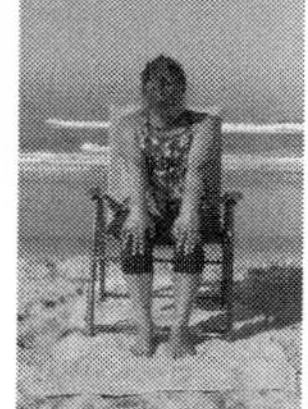
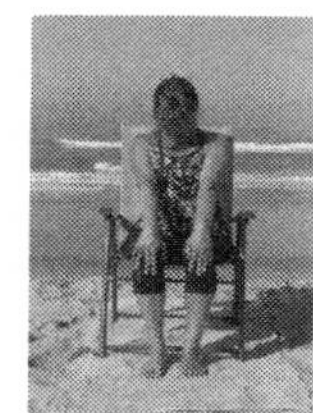
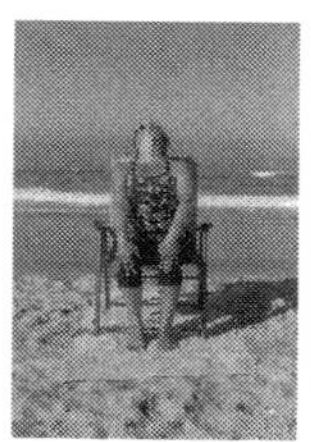
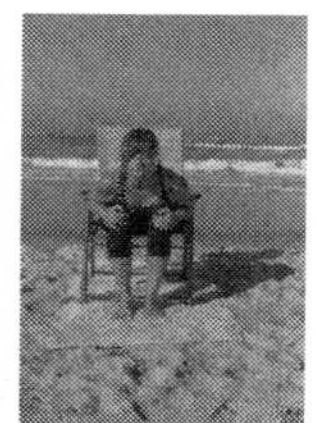

Triangle Posture/Trikonasana

Begin with your hands at your sides, breathing in through your nose and out through the center of your lips. Take three breaths. Now rest your palms on your thighs.

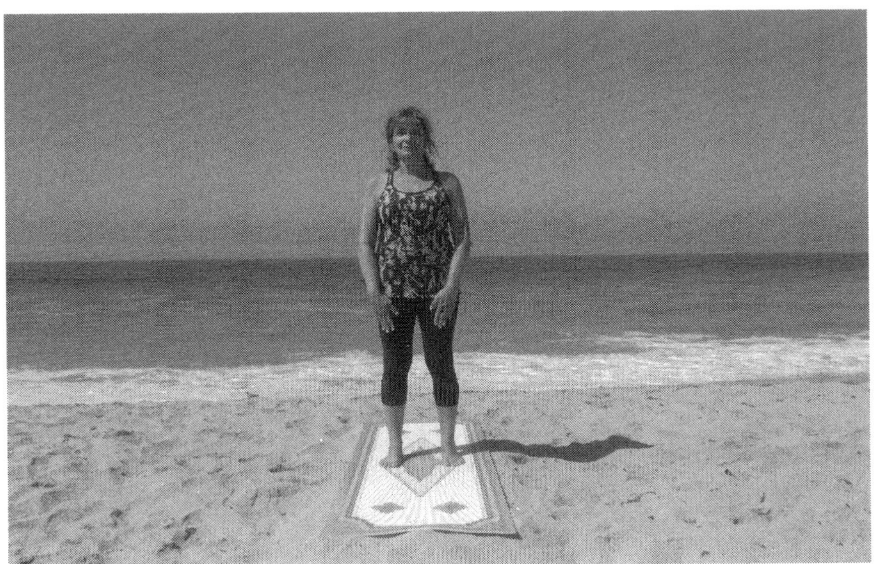

As you are breathing in bring straight arms up at shoulder level parallel to the ground, with the palms facing down and go up onto your toes. As you're breathing out, turn to your upper body and arms to your left. Once your arms are pointing to the left bring your heels on the ground. Breathe in.

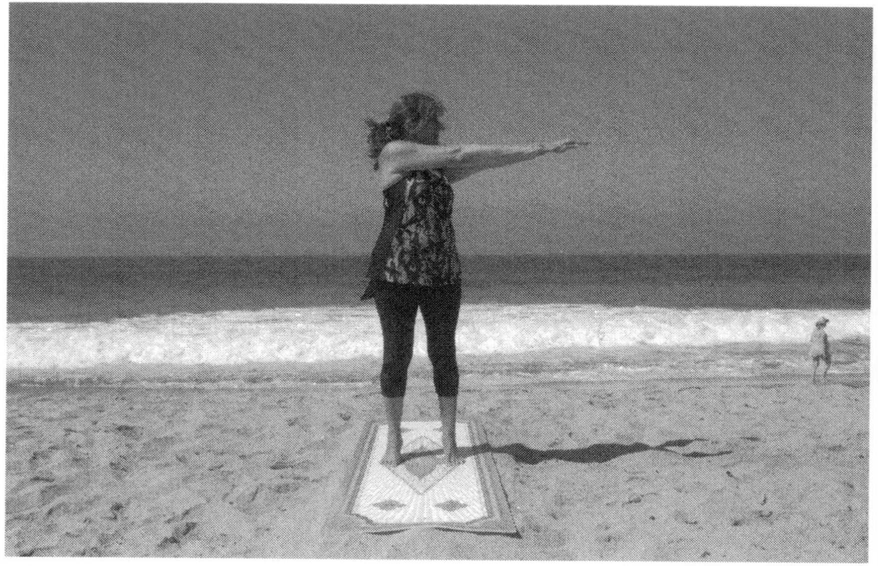

As you breathe out take your right palm and run it along the inside of your right thigh and calf and go down until you place your hand as close to the ground as possible. Your left arm is straight and pointing toward the sky with your fingertips relaxed. Turn your head as if you were looking at your left hand. Stay in this position for three breaths Then come out of the pose in the reverse order- taking your right palm along your right inner calf and thigh and straightening your body up as you're breathing in. Left arm goes down at your side and both arms hang at your sides.

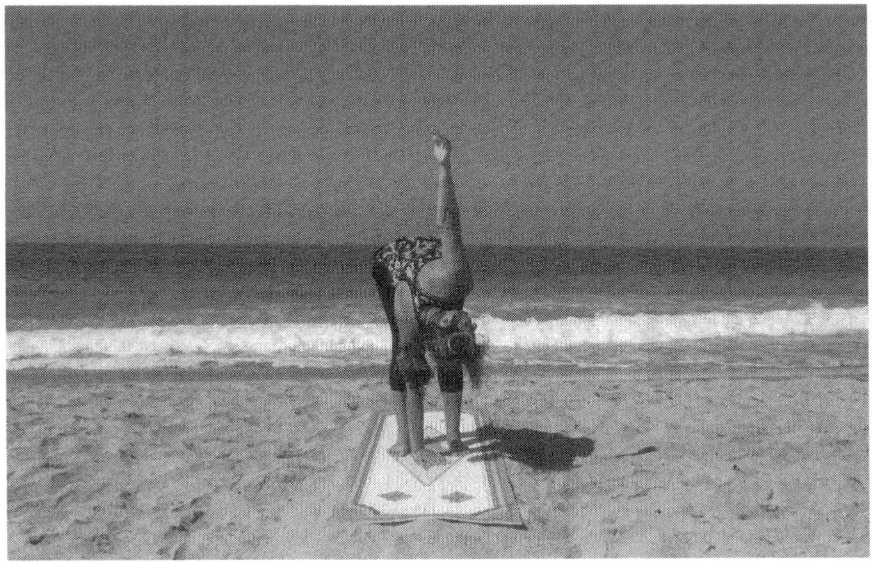

Rest for a few breaths and do the exact sequence of movements, but this time turning your upper body to the right and bringing the left arm along the inside of the left leg and the right arm up.

Modified triangle posture

While Sitting - Begin with your arms at your side breathing in through your nose and out through the center of your lips. Take three breaths. Now rest your palms on your thighs.

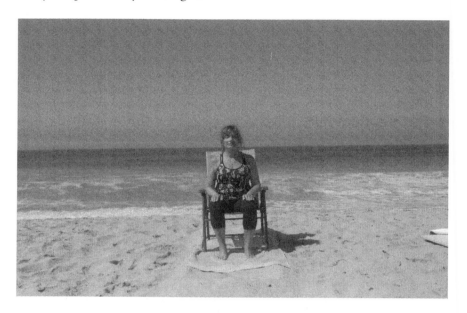

As you are breathing in, bring straight arms up at shoulder level parallel to the ground with the palms facing the ground. As you're breathing out, turn to your upper body and arms to your left.

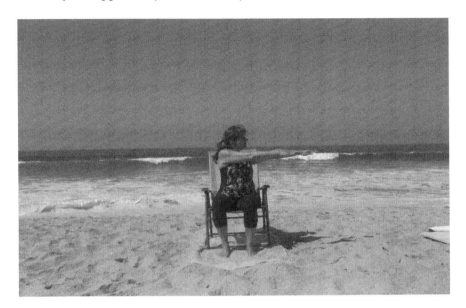

While sitting -As you breathe out take your right palm and run it along the inside of your right thigh and calf and go down until you place your hand as close to the ground as possible. Your left arm is straight and pointing toward the sky with your fingertips relaxed. Turn your head as if you were looking at your left hand. Stay in this position for three breaths Then come out of the pose in the reverse order- taking your right palm along your right inner calf and thigh and straightening your body up as you're breathing in. Left arm goes down at your side and both arms hang at your sides.

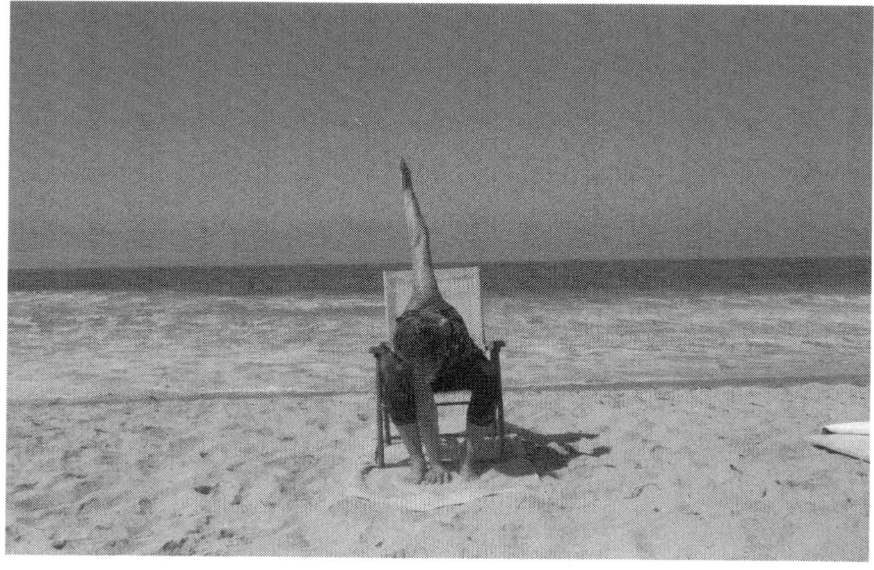

Rest for a few breaths and do the exact sequence of movements turning the right side of your body and placing the left hand on the ground an the right arm up.

CHAPTER 15

Breath

Breath is our life source. The importance of it can't be stressed enough. Although you have been breathing your whole life, it's important that you breathe as your body is meant to breathe. Our bodies are meant to take full, nourishing breaths in a relaxed and natural way. This changes when we have tension in our bodies. When we are afraid or stressed, our breathing becomes shallow. If you have been spending much of your life with stress, you are breathing with shallow breaths most of the time. In addition to that, keeping in the stomach area has become a habit for many of us and that certainly makes it so you can't take a deep, full breath. Old habits need to be changed to bring the body back to health.

At this point, you will learn what the most nourishing, healthy way of breathing is for you. Follow the guidelines in the subsequent pages closely. Move from step to step at your own pace and in your own time. Progressing faster is not better. Progressing gently and naturally is best. Your body will determine when to move on to the next step. Only move forward when you are performing that particular breath spontaneously and with ease. They're all building blocks. In order for your structure to be sound and stable, each block needs to be strong and capable of holding the blocks that will be built upon them. Be aware of every step and enjoy the process.

Step 1 Foundation Breath

Before we begin, it's important you know the correct way to breathe. When you inhale your stomach should be filling up, and when you exhale your stomach should be going in. Think of your stomach as a balloon. What happens to a balloon when you blow air into it? It expands. The same principal applies to your stomach area. And as the air is leaving the stomach it deflates in the same way a balloon does.

Sit up straight and take a breath. Observe what happens. If your stomach is getting bigger as you are breathing in, then that's a good sign. It means you're doing it correctly. If your stomach is deflating or remaining the same while you inhale, then try to breathe as I have told you. If it's still not clear, then try the following:

Lie down on your back. Breathe as you naturally would. Observe what is happening. Observe how your stomach moves up as you inhale and down as you exhale. This is the natural way your body wants to breathe. That is how you need to breathe when you are sitting or standing. Technically, what you are feeling is your diaphragm, the breath is not going to your belly, but in order for you to have a full breath, that is how it feels.

For the next week I want you to simply be aware of your breath until you are comfortable breathing in the way I've described. Make sure you are following this process. Until you are comfortable breathing like this, please don't proceed to any of the following breaths. This is the basic foundation for your breath, and although it seems simple, it does take time to create this habit in yourself. Even if you have already been breathing this way, please continue to do so, but now I want you to observe your breath throughout the day. Find enjoyment in taking your focus to your breath.

In addition to this form of breathing, as you inhale focus on taking air in through your nose instead of your mouth. As you exhale, make a small "O"" with your lips and breathe out through the center of your lips. Take deep, slow and gentle breaths in, and breathe out using the same control. You will find that not only will you start breathing properly; your body and mind will begin slowing down to a relaxed state. The temples on the side of your head begin relaxing when your breath releases through the center of your lips.

Ideally, do this at least three times a day. Take at least 20 breaths, in the morning, in the afternoon, and in the evening before bed. You may choose to do it more often, and that would be terrific! Initially, if it's easier for you to lie down to practice Step 1, do so. But, after two days, do this sitting or standing. It's important you eventually breathe like this at all times. Practice makes you better at it. Practice will also lead to it becoming automatic. Let this become an integrated part of you.

Now you have spent a minimum of two weeks with this breath, practicing several times a day. You have reached a point of comfort and ease with this breath and are ready to move on. Go on to Step 2. If you find you need to go back to Step 1 for any reason, please don't hesitate to do so.

Step 2 Yogic Breath-Inhalation

Once you have become comfortable with breathing correctly, you can learn yogic breath. This entails filling your lungs fully and completely. Begin your breath by filling your stomach, then fill your chest, and finally take your breath into your upper chest toward your shoulders. Don't try to lift the shoulders; they will lift naturally. Practice breathing this way three times each day. Take at least 20 breaths. Do this in the same manner you did when you were learning to breathe correctly. Become mindful of your breath as it fills your lungs. Breathe in through your nose and out through the center of your lips. Practice this for at least one week. If at the week's end you are not comfortable breathing this way, then continue practicing daily until you are. Take as long as you need. The most important part is for you to be effortless in doing it. Remember these breaths are building blocks. Don't move on to the next breath until you have integrated Steps 1 and 2 and are comfortable practicing it.

Step 3 Yogic Breath with Exhalation

You have now spent some time focusing on full, proper inhalation, so now let's incorporate proper exhalation. As you breathe in, you are filling the stomach, chest and shoulders, and now as you breathe out, do so in the opposite order. As you are breathing out, release the breath from the shoulder area, then the chest and finally the stomach. Do this slowly, gently, and uniformly. Observe the process and be aware as it's happening. Practice this for at least a week three times a day, taking at least 20 breaths each time. If you find that you would like to take more breaths, by all means do so. There is no limit to how many breaths to take. This practice will bring you much balance and wellness. It is very important to your total wellbeing. It may not be easy initially, but I have no doubt you will get it once you practice. The main point is that you be with your breath. Be aware of what parts are filling with the breath and then what parts are releasing the breath. Do it systematically. What will happen is that you will find yourself spontaneously doing it with no effort. I can't stress enough how important this is.

Now you are ready to guide your breath and use it to energize, balance and heal you. Pranayama guided breath will be a very important part of your healing process. The ability to bring harmony to your mind and body through your breath will benefit you tremendously. It will be what helps your body come into alignment and heal. Please don't underestimate how powerful guiding your energy breath is.

Nadishodan Pranayama

Alternate Nostril Breathing

The most important pranayama you will learn is Nadishodan. It is the process of breathing alternately through your nostrils. This breath is truly the most important component in this whole book. It will balance your nervous system, bringing balance to your mind, body and whole being. In order to heal, physical and mental balance needs to take place.

Follow the steps below:

1. Using your right hand, place your index and middle finger in the space between your eyebrows. These will be your anchors. As you breathe in, press down gently with those fingers, and as you breathe out lift them slightly. Do this for five breaths, focusing and being aware of that spot between your brows. Inhale and exhale through both nostrils.

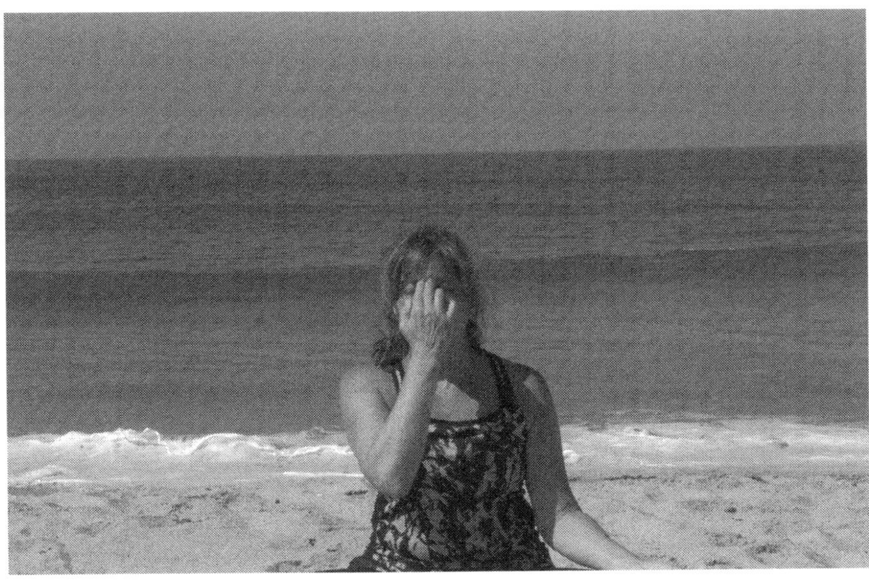

2. Leave your index and middle fingers in place; pressings gently, and now take your thumb and press gently on the side of your right nostril to close it. Breathe in through your left nostril and breathe

out through your left nostril. Do this for five slow, smooth and uniform breaths.

3. Lift your thumb and now press your left nostril with your ring finger so that you block the airflow. Breathe in and out through your right nostril. Do this for five slow, smooth and uniform breaths.

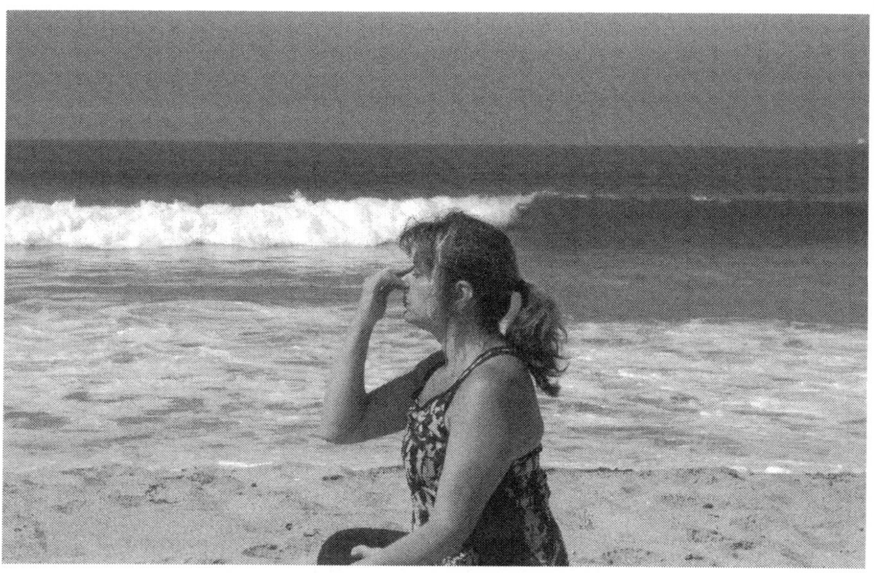

Now bring your thumb onto the right nostril and breathe in through the left nostril. Cover the left nostril with your ring finger, lift the thumb and breathe out through your right nostril, and then breathe in through the right nostril. Lift your ring finger bringing the thumb down on the right nostril, and breathe out through the left nostril. Breathe in through the left nostril and repeat the process all over again, alternating nostrils slowly, gently and uniformly. There is no hurry in doing this. Do this for five complete rounds: in through the left, out through the right, in through the right, out through the left.

4. Then drop your hand and breathe in and out slowly through both nostrils. Allow yourself to become aware of your breath.

5. For three days, practice this three times each day, morning, afternoon and evening before bed. Do five repetitions of this each time.
6. Starting on the fourth day, begin doing 11 repetitions of this practice three times a day, morning, afternoon and evening before bed. Continue doing this every day. I recommend you continue this practice every single day, even after you become well. The benefits you'll receive from this will go well beyond what any supplement can offer.

Bhramari Pranayama

Wasps Buzzing

This form of pranayama is excellent for your brain. It will bring vibration to the brain and this is very desirable, as we want our brains to exercise as much as possible. Through this breath you will be doing exactly that. There are different ways of exercising the brain. One way is by learning something new, and in this way creating new pathways in the brain. The other is by causing subtle vibration in the brain. When you exercise physically your brain starts growing new neurons. Once you stop exercising, these neurons will die if you don't stimulate them by exercising the brain. It's important that you create new neurons and set new pathways in any way you can. Through Bhramari, you will be activating any new neurons to continue to grow through vibration. I recommend that after you practice your yoga postures/asanas, you sit quietly and perform Bhramari immediately afterward. Yoga is, in fact, a form of physical exercise. You can also do this immediately after doing any other kind of physical exercise. The point is to stimulate the brain so that your new neurons continue to grow. Below is a step-by-step guide to practicing Bhramari.

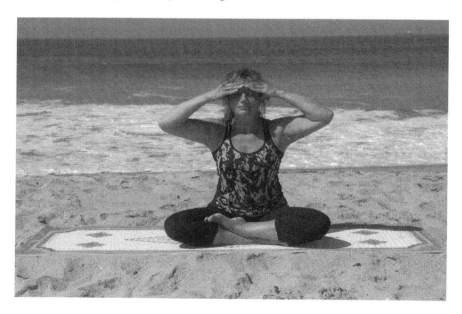

1. Sit in a comfortable position with your back straight yet relaxed. Your neck and head are also straight and relaxed.
2. Bring your middle fingers to the center of your forehead, with the tips touching each other.
3. At the same time, place your thumbs over the portion of your outer ear above the ear canal and press down on it so it covers the ear canal. Make sure your ear canal is covered so that outside noises become muffled.
4. Take a deep breath through your nose.
5. As you breath out purse your lips together and make the sound of wasps buzzing or humming. In truth, it should sound a lot more like bees buzzing than wasps. Do this so that you can hear it inside your head. Feel the vibration inside your head.
6. Do this 11 times and then put your hands in your lap. Rest your left palm in your right palm with both facing the sky. Let your thumbs gently touch each other.
7. Sit in silence for a few minutes. Listen to the subtle sound of the humming as if it's coming from a distance, leading to deeper silence. Allow the body and mind to be still. Let the brain absorb the stimulation it has been given in total relaxation.

This is an extremely effective breath for bringing new life to the brain. It is also very good for calming anxiety and depression. It has quite a calming and relaxing overall effect on the whole body and mind. Only when the body is relaxed does it have the opportunity to heal. Allow yourself to have that. Give yourself the gift of relaxation.

Both of the pranayama you are learning are very important components of your healing process. Practice Bhramari immediately after you have practiced your asanas.

Continue practicing both of these breathing techniques with full confidence and awareness. If at any time during the day you feel the need to practice these for a few minutes, don't hesitate to do so. There is nothing in these breaths that can hurt you. On the contrary, they can do nothing but help you. With practice, you'll begin feeling the ways they will bring about change in your total well being.

CHAPTER 16

Meditation

The third part of the process is meditation. Please keep in mind there is no strict goal in any of these processes. Each will progress at it's own pace. But, it is essential that you practice all three every day. If for some reason you have to miss a day, just pick it right back up the next day. Please don't ever feel pressure or stress in your practice. Try to live by the suggestions in the earlier chapters and know this will give you life and health. Now, let's talk about what meditation is.

Meditation is not something you "do." It's simply a calming of the mind. You can think of it in terms of giving the mind a break. There is no right or wrong meditation experience. Your experience is yours alone, and someone else may have a totally different one. It's subjective and indescribable because it's quite a personal process unique to you. That being said, I will teach you techniques to help your mind focus and release the thoughts that come and go, and as a result, you will have the tools to reach a state of mental relaxation.

The most important part I want you to understand before we begin is that it's okay to have thoughts as you are trying to sit in silence. Acknowledge your thoughts, be aware of them, then step back mentally and release them. Be an observer of your thoughts; don't become involved in them. Just observe as they come and as they go without judgment and without reaction. Become mindful of the process, and then you can move beyond your thoughts.

Centering

Before you begin any part of your practice, take time to find your center. It will enhance and enrich your experience. This is because you are focusing on the "now," the moment in time in which you have chosen to spend nurturing and healing yourself. In coming into the "now," you will be able to more clearly move through your practice in a spontaneous, relaxed and mindful manner. The whole point of centering is to bring you to an effortless state at the present moment and leave any other thoughts or emotions aside. It will help calm the mind and align your whole being in order to be more receptive to a few minutes of silence.

Below is a sequence you can follow to center yourself. It is also available on transcendingms.com:

Sit in a comfortable position. Have your back straight yet relaxed. Have your neck and head straight yet relaxed as well. Breathe in through your nose and out through the center of your lips. Do this at the pace your body naturally dictates. Don't try to impose a rhythm; follow your own body's breathing rhythm. Place your hands in your lap with palms facing toward the sky. Hold the left hand in the right with thumbs gently touching each other. Become aware of the ground below you. Feel which parts of your body touch the earth. Become aware of the temperature of the space you're in. Is your left knee in balance with your right knee? Is your left shoulder in balance with the right? Don't adjust them, just be aware of them. Notice the sounds around you. Now become aware of sounds in the distance. Be aware of the taste in your mouth. No judgment, just be aware. Now, as you breathe in, notice any fragrances in the air around you. Simply observe. And, finally, even though your eyes are closed, what do you see in the space behind your forehead? Imagine this space as a movie screen where images can be projected upon it. Now take your awareness to your mind. Pay attention to any thoughts coming and going through it. Don't try to stop these thoughts, just observe them. Now, become aware that all of this is happening in this moment in time—the "now." Yesterday was made of "nows" and tomorrow will be made of "nows." Each moment is "now." Be aware that now you are safe. Now you are breathing. Now you have thoughts that are coming and going. And now be aware that your thoughts are simply that—thoughts. They're transient. They're temporary. They are not you. As you breathe in, be aware of the effect these thoughts have on your body and the effect your body has on these thoughts, and let the two become one in this process. Let your awareness go to the essential way your mind and body are not only connected, but are one.

Now that you've centered your body and your mind, take your attention to the spot in the center of your chest at heart level. As you inhale, begin to breathe in through the place in your chest, and as you are breathing out, do so through this same place. Slowly and deliberately, with awareness, breathe in and out through the center of your chest—your heart space. As you breathe in, fill your heart with the energy that comes with your breath, and as you exhale release the energy and notice any tension leaving your body. Breathe in again and fill your heart space with peaceful energy. Breathe out and release any fear slowly and gently. Breathe in and fill your heart with strength; breathe out and release any sadness. Breathe in and fill your heart with joy; breathe out and release any tension, anger, or any other feelings causing you disharmony. Breathe in with harmony, balance and love. Let your heart be filled with love and gratitude for the moment you have been granted, and use it to nurture, heal and, above all, love yourself and those around you. Breathe in and feel the balance and harmony in your heart, in your mind and in your body. All three becoming one. All three aware and centered in this beautiful moment in time.

You can practice this at any time of day, but be sure to always do so before practicing your asanas (postures). Also, prior to beginning your focusing technique for meditation it is a good idea to do this centering exercise as well. It only takes a few minutes, but the benefits you will reap will make a huge difference in your overall practice.

When learning to meditate, a focusing technique is vital in silencing the mind. When focusing on a word or a mental image, your mind can potentially block all other thoughts and lead you to a place of mental, physical and spiritual peace. Beginning your meditation practice with guided meditations is another effective way to ease into quieting your mind until you become more familiar with the process. Pick a time of day when you don't have something you're obligated to do or somewhere you must be soon after. Set a timer for your meditations. In this way, your mind won't wonder how long you have been doing it or whether it's time to stop. Begin with two minutes, then when you feel the need to go longer, set the timer for three, and continue adding minutes as you progress. There is no right or wrong length of time to meditate, so take it slowly. You will eventually reach a point when you won't need a timer any longer. After practicing daily for some time, what you will find is that you won't need to rely on guided meditations anymore, and your own inner voice will guide you in your process.

Focusing Techniques

SoHum

SoHum is a focusing technique using a mantra. A mantra is a word you say silently to yourself while focusing. You will be focusing on the mantra with the breath.

Sit comfortably. Your back is straight, your neck is straight, your head is straight and they are all relaxed. Put your palms in your lap with the right palm holding the left and both facing the sky with thumbs gently touching each other. Begin breathing in and out slowly, gently and uniformly. Breathe in through your nose and out through the center of your lips. Focus your awareness on your breath as it enters your body and as it leaves your body. Let this happen without effort. Continue doing this for five breaths. Now when you breathe in, mentally say "SO." As you breathe out, mentally say "HUM." In "SO," out "HUM." Do this for 11 breaths. Don't worry if you lose count, just keep the focus on the SO HUM as you breathe. Gently release the mantra and stay where you are in silence for as long as you like, releasing all thoughts. If thoughts come, acknowledge them and tell them you will address them later, but don't entertain them. Most importantly, do not try to suppress them. Let life flow through you. When you feel you are ready to come out of the meditation, whether it's two minutes or 20 minutes, take five deep, full yogic breaths with gratitude. Remember, gratitude seals the deal. If you find that initially you are restless and fidgety, don't worry, it's to be expected. Your mind isn't used to being quiet and may want to fight it. Keep at it and the stillness will come. Know that all meditations will be different. There is no right or wrong way and no good or bad meditation practice. There are moments when our minds are merely busier than others. This is your own personal journey. Just make sure it's always made with deep gratitude.

Anapana

Anapana is a focusing technique using your breath. You will experience the breath as it's coming into the body and as it's leaving the body. It's a very effective way of concentrating and sharpening the mind, which will lead to silencing it.

Sit comfortably. Your back is straight, your neck is straight, your head is straight and they are all relaxed. Put your palms in your lap with the right palm holding the left and both facing the sky with thumbs gently touching each other. Begin slowly breathing in through the nose and out through the center of the lips, gently and uniformly. Let the breath guide you; don't try to control it. After five breaths, begin breathing in through the nose and out through the nose. Again, let the breath be your guide. Now let your focus go to your nostrils. As you're breathing in, be aware of the breath entering through your nostrils, and as you're breathing out feel the breath leaving through your nostrils and brushing the area between your upper lip and nose. Continue breathing and focusing on the breath going in and the breath going out. Feel how cool the breath going in is and how much warmer the breath going out is. Focus only on the breath. If and when your mind drifts away from the process, gently bring it back to your breath. Allow the breath to flow and simply be an observer of how it feels at the nostril area. There will come a time when you will feel full mental relaxation and well being through this practice. When ready to come out of the process, take five full yogic breaths with gratitude.

Both of these focusing techniques are very effective. You can choose to practice either one on any given day. My suggestion would be to choose one technique and practice it consistently and exclusively for at least two weeks. Then do the same with the other technique. In this way, you can feel the progression of your practice with each. It's up to you which technique you choose to eventually use on a daily basis, or you might decide to do both. For now, practice only one daily, but feel free to use it as often as you like.

In Conclusion

Then What?

So as you apply all the suggestions in this book I need you to think about something. Once you are well, once you are strong, once you are symptom free... then what?

Then what? What will you choose to do with the gift you have been given? What will you do with that second chance you now have? What will you do after transcending?

Think about this and think about it without stress or worry but rather with an open heart. Why did you get sick in the first place? Maybe going back to the way things were before you got sick is not a good idea. Maybe you should think about adopting your new found tools and ways permanently.

OK, so you do this. Then what? What will you do with this new found way? Will you remember that the receiving is in the giving? Will you remember to be grateful every day for all that you have and all that you are? Will you remember to pass along this opportunity you have been given to others? Will you remember that it is in this way that you will continue to heal and transcend yourself? Will you remember that love is where it all heals? Love for yourself of course, but also the world around you. I am not asking you to make yourself responsible for others, but I am asking you to make yourself a vehicle to help where you can and to give of yourself with love and gratitude in your heart. Remember, gratitude seals the deal.

Remember to enrich your spirit by truly living in gratitude every day, every moment throughout the day. Let it become your habit and your way of being. What better way to live could there be?... Then what? Then that...

I wish you ease, harmony, and balance and above all I wish for you a life filled with love.

31 Day Journey to Peace

The 31 Day Journey to Peace is meant to give you a daily roadmap to bring peace to your life. It is a very simple process. A different step every day to take you to balance, harmony and ease. You will be taking yourself toward that state of being one small step at a time for 31 days. Enjoy the journey…

1st day-

Before you go to sleep tonight take 10 full breaths with your eyes closed. Breathe in through your nose and breathe out through your lips.

Try to do it slowly and gently. Ease yourself into a state of relaxation.

Sweet dreams…

2nd day-

Tonight, before you go to sleep, take 10 full breaths sitting up, with your back straight. Put one hand on your chest and one hand on your abdomen. As you inhale, the hand on the abdomen should rise more than the hand on the chest. As you exhale, slowly bring your abdomen in to exhale as much air as possible. Focus on your breath, breathing in through your nose and out through the lips, slowly and gently. Ease yourself into a state of relaxation.

Sweet dreams…

3rd day-

When you wake up today, take ten breaths with your eyes closed, sitting up with a straight back. Place one hand on your chest and one on your abdomen, the way you did the night before. Focus on your breath and the beauty of being alive today. Feel the calmness with which you will start your day today.

Enjoy your day...

Tonight, before you go to sleep, do the same, and as you focus on your breath, focus on the beauty of your breath and in gratitude feel the life force within you. Ease yourself into a state of relaxation and gratitude.

Sweet dreams...

4th day-

Today, let it be a day of giving. A small gesture, but with a tremendous impact. Please take a bag, it can be whatever kind of bag you choose. Fill it with items that a person in need could use. It can be food, a toothbrush and toothpaste, or maybe even writing materials, or all of the above. Fill it with whatever YOUR heart desires to give. Then take it with you when you leave your house. Give it to a homeless person or any person in need. My only request is that you give it to a stranger, someone you don't know. If you're sick and can't leave the house, fill it and give it to someone else to pass it on for you. You will both benefit from this…

Enjoy your day…

Also, continue today with your 10 breaths in the morning and your ten breaths in the evening. Let them help you begin your day in peace and end your day in gratitude…

Sweet dreams…

5th day-

Let's lift someone's spirit today. Without going out of your way to do so, say something unexpectedly nice to someone. It may be someone you know and love, or it may be a stranger in a store. But it has to be genuine. Meaning, you must mean it. For example, if you see someone who is wearing a dress you like, tell them how pretty their dress is. If you don't think the dress is pretty, then don't say it. Above all, be genuine in what you say…

Enjoy your day…

Also continue today with your 10 breaths in the morning and your ten breaths in the evening. Let them help you begin your day in peace and end your day with gratitude…

Sweet dreams…

6th day-

The past couple of days have been about making a difference in someone else. Today, take at least 90 minutes for yourself. What would you like to do with those 90 minutes? What would make your heart full? Only you know what that is. It can be as simple as sitting with a cup of tea or coffee on the beach or a park. Be kind to yourself today…

Enjoy your day…

Also continue today with your 10 breaths in the morning and your ten breaths in the evening. Let them help you begin your day in peace and end your day with gratitude…

Sweet dreams…

7th day-

We are adding one more step to your breaths today. When you wake up, take 10 full breaths sitting up, with your back straight. Put one hand on your chest and one hand on your abdomen. As you inhale slowly through your nose, the hand on the abdomen should rise more than the hand on the chest. At the end of your inhalation, take a moment to pause before you begin your exhalation. As you exhale slowly through your lips, gently bring your abdomen in to exhale as much air as possible. Focus on your breath and the beauty of being alive today. Be aware of how important you are. Feel the calmness with which you will start your day today.

Enjoy your day...

Tonight, before you go to sleep, do the same, and as you focus on your breath, focus on the beauty of your breath and in gratitude feel the life force within you. Be aware of all the miracles you witnessed today. Ease yourself into a state of relaxation and gratitude.

Sweet dreams…

8th day-

As you take your breaths this morning, make sure that you have your eyes gently closed, if you haven't been doing so already. Take 10 full breaths sitting up, with your back straight. Place your palms in your lap with the right palm supporting the left one and facing the sky and your thumbs gently touching each other. As you inhale slowly through your nose, the abdomen should rise more than the chest. At the end of your inhalation, take a moment to pause before you begin your exhalation. As you exhale slowly through your lips, gently bring your abdomen in to exhale as much air as possible. Focus on your breath and the beauty of being alive today. Focus on this moment in time with every breath. Feel the calmness with which you will start your day today...

Enjoy you day...

Tonight, before you go to sleep, do the same, and as you focus on your breath, focus on the beauty of your breath and in gratitude feel the life force within you. Focus on this moment in time and how safe you are. Ease yourself into a state of relaxation and gratitude. As you do, take time to give thanks for at least one specific moment of today.

Sweet dreams…

9th day-

Today, be aware of using the word "should". Stop for a moment when you find yourself saying or thinking it, and try to replace it with "need to", "have to" or "want to". If you can't replace it, then why are you doing it? You have no desire in whatever that is. If your heart isn't in it, then don't. Try to eliminate "should" from your vocabulary today. Allow "you" to be genuine.

Begin and end your day with 10 breaths and intentions as yesterday, in this way-

As you take your breaths this morning, make sure that you have your eyes gently closed, if you haven't been doing so already. Take 10 full breaths sitting up, with your back straight. Place your palms in your lap with the right palm supporting the left one and facing the sky and your thumbs gently touching each other. As you inhale slowly through your nose, the abdomen should rise more than the chest. At the end of your inhalation, take a moment to pause before you begin your exhalation. As you exhale slowly through your lips, gently bring your abdomen in to exhale as much air as possible. Focus on your breath and the beauty of being alive today. Focus on this moment in time with every breath. Feel the calmness with which you will start your day today...

Enjoy your day...

Tonight, before you go to sleep, do the same, and as you focus on your breath, focus on the beauty of your breath and in gratitude feel the life force within you. Focus on this moment in time and how safe you are. Ease yourself into a state of relaxation and gratitude. As you do, take time to give thanks for at least one specific moment of today.

Sweet dreams…

10th day-

Trying to not sound repetitive, but what you did yesterday, in all ways is so important, it needs to be repeated today. Let yourself settle into a life without "should."

Today, be aware of using the word "should." Stop for a moment when you find yourself saying or thinking it, and try to replace it with "need to," "have to" or "want to." If you can't replace it, then why are you doing it? You have no desire in whatever that is. If your heart isn't in it, then don't. Try to eliminate "should" from your vocabulary today. Allow "you" to be genuine.

As you take your breaths this morning, make sure that you have your eyes gently closed, if you haven't been doing so already. Take 10 full breaths sitting up, with your back straight. Place your palms in your lap with the right palm supporting the left one and facing the sky and your thumbs gently touching each other. As you inhale slowly through your nose, the abdomen should rise more than the chest. At the end of your inhalation, take a moment to pause before you begin your exhalation. As you exhale slowly through your lips, gently bring your abdomen in to exhale as much air as possible. Focus on your breath and the beauty of being alive today. Focus on this moment in time with every breath. Feel the calmness with which you will start your day today…

Enjoy you day...

Tonight, before you go to sleep, do the same, and as you focus on your breath, focus on the beauty of your breath and in gratitude feel the life force within you. Focus on this moment in time and how safe you are. Ease yourself into a state of relaxation and gratitude. As you do, take time to give thanks for at least two specific moments of today.

Sweet dreams…

11th day-

Today would be a good day to get in touch with someone you love, who you haven't talked to in a while. Maybe you've just let time pass by, but take a moment to call them. Texting doesn't count. It's important that you talk to them and tell them how much you love them. Don't call because you should, call because you want to... Feel the power of love...

Continue with your morning breaths and evening breaths as you have for the past two days. Please do those faithfully. Don't underestimate the power they have in this process. For your convenience, they are below as a reference.

As you take your breaths this morning, make sure that you have your eyes gently closed, if you haven't been doing so already. Take 10 full breaths sitting up, with your back straight. Place your palms in your lap with the right palm supporting the left one and facing the sky and your thumbs gently touching each other. As you inhale slowly through your nose, the abdomen should rise more than the chest. At the end of your inhalation, take a moment to pause before you begin your exhalation. As you exhale slowly through your lips, gently bring your abdomen in to exhale as much air as possible. Focus on your breath and the beauty of being alive today. Focus on this moment in time with every breath. Feel the calmness with which you will start your day today…

Enjoy you day...

Tonight, before you go to sleep, do the same, and as you focus on your breath, focus on the beauty of your breath and in gratitude feel the life force within you. Focus on this moment in time and how safe you are. Ease yourself into a state of relaxation and gratitude. As you do, take time to give thanks for at least two specific moments of today.

Sweet dreams…

12th day-

Acceptance vs. expectations is the focus for today. Allow yourself to accept events today as they come to you. Release any kind of expectation. Observe yourself when expecting someone to behave the way YOU want them to. Consciously stop yourself and truly make an effort to accept them for who they are and what their choices are. Apply this to all situations today with awareness. In the same way you let go of "should," let go of expectations and allow yourself to accept others and life events as they develop. Enjoy the surprises that will come up and the simplicity of being open to life.

As you take your 10 breaths this morning, with your eyes gently closed, check that you are sitting up, with your back straight but relaxed. Place your palms in your lap with the right palm supporting the left one and facing the sky and your thumbs gently touching each other. As you inhale slowly through your nose, the abdomen should rise more than the chest. At the end of your inhalation, take a moment to pause before you begin your exhalation. As you exhale slowly through your lips, gently bring your abdomen in to exhale as much air as possible. Focus on accepting this moment in time with every breath. Feel the calmness with which you will start your day today...

Enjoy you day...

Tonight, before you go to sleep, do the same, and as you focus on your breath, focus on the beauty of acceptance. Ease yourself into a state of relaxation and gratitude. As you do, take time to give thanks for at least two specific moments of today in which you were able to release all expectations and accept. Feel the freedom that comes with it...

Sweet dreams…

13th day-

The one constant in this process has been your 10 breaths in the morning and in the evening. You now know how to breathe the way your body is intended to breathe and with it your body relaxes and releases stress.

In the morning, before you begin your 10 breaths today, think of 3 reasons to be grateful. Then begin your breaths. Feel the difference gratitude makes in you as you finish your breaths.

Give yourself at least 90 minutes today to do something which your heart really wants. It's your choice. Be kind to yourself without any sense of guilt. It's important that you love yourself and honor who you are. Try to go through your day with ease in that love.

Enjoy your day...

Tonight, before you begin your breaths, think over your day and 3 reasons on this day for which you're grateful. Let your sleep be filled with gratitude and love for all you are and all you are blessed with.

Sweet dreams...

14th day-

A brand new week and a brand new day. Take a moment this morning to be grateful for 3 things about yourself. There is no right or wrong answer to this. It's personal, and as such, only you know what those are.

Then, begin your ten breaths today in gratitude for you and who you are. As you inhale and exhale be aware of the miracle of your body.

Make a point today to be aware of any self criticism. If you find that you are putting yourself down mentally, shift the thought. If you find yourself saying it out loud, shift the thought. Make a point of being as kind to yourself, as you would be to a small child. You deserve no less than that.

Enjoy your day...

Tonight, before you begin your 10 breaths, mentally go over your day and bring to mind 3 moments today for which you are grateful that you are you. While having your ten breaths, let your awareness settle in that gratitude and allow your body and mind to relax.

Sweet dreams...

15th day-

I hope you found out yesterday just how remarkable you are. Today, I want you to take that remarkable being a step further.

Go through your day with personal excellence. No matter what you do, do it to the best of your ability, without comparing yourself with anyone. Bring your genuine self into everything you do. Even in your "hello, how are you" to others, mean it. Only you can give what you have to give, in the way you and only you, would give it. Know, that the world around you is a better place as a result.

Continue your 10 breaths this morning. Between your inhalation and exhalation pause and let the gratitude for "you" settle in to every breath. Let the understanding of the importance of you, be part of you, without a doubt as you start your day.

Enjoy your day...

Tonight, before you begin your breaths, go over the day in your mind. Recall 3 moments in which you felt personal excellence in what you were doing. Allow gratitude to settle in, for the ability to perform the way you do, in being you. Begin the 10 breaths, breathing in through your nose, pause in humble gratitude, and exhale through the lips. Let your sleep be filled with love for the being that you are and gratitude for being you.

Sweet dreams…

16th day-

Although I seem to be focusing on the other aspects of your days, please know how important it is to continue to take the time for your 10 breaths in the morning and at night. It's that moment with the breath, which will continue to make a difference in you, no matter what your days are like.

This morning, before you begin, say "thank you" out loud. Let the meaning of those words settle into the space between your inhalations and exhalations and permeate every cell in your body as you take the ten breaths.

Enjoy your day...

"Compare" is the word for today. As your day unfolds today, catch yourself comparing, mentally as well as out loud. Shift your thoughts when this happens. Let your personal excellence take over any thought of comparing. What other people do or have, is of no consequence to you. Be aware of what you need, not what you think you should have or be. Live from your heart, not from fear of lacking, and watch how that energy will give to you what your heart wants. Be willing and ready to receive it. Allow yourself to receive.

Tonight, before you begin your breaths, think of 3 things for which your personal excellence opened the door for you to receive. Again, out loud say "thank you." Let the meaning of those words settle into the space between your inhalations and exhalations and permeate every cell in your body as you take the ten breaths. Let your sleep be filled with gratitude and love for who you are.

Sweet dreams…

17th day-

You have become aware of comparing... Now, I would like you to be aware of complaining; mentally as well as out loud. When you find yourself complaining, shift your thoughts. Focus on what you have, not what you don't have. Gratitude, gratitude, gratitude.

Before you begin your breaths this morning, say "thank you" silently. Greet today with those words. Let them settle in the space between your inhalations and exhalations.

Enjoy your day...

Tonight, think of 3 moments today in which you were totally present. As you breathe, be aware of the present moment of each breath during all 10 breaths. Let gratitude settle in for all you have and all you are at this moment in time.

Sweet dreams…

18th day-

On to the third "C" which troubles the mind.

Control.

Today, allow your 10 breaths to just happen with your eyes closed. As you're breathing, observe how your body is naturally breathing without any guidance whatsoever. Feel the freedom in letting the breaths flow in their natural state.

Enjoy your day...

Trying to control situations and people can be a source of stress. Today, be aware of your need to control. Be open to the way other people may think a situation, project or challenge can be performed or resolved. Be open to allowing those close to you to go through their day today, without trying to tell them how. When you feel the need to "take over" or "advise", let it go and shift your thoughts to allowing others to grow. Watch them blossom and feel the freedom it will not only give them, but you as well.

Before beginning your 10 breaths tonight, take a moment to recall an instance in which you released your need to control today. How did it feel? The lightness that comes with allowing others to grow will have a very beautiful effect for all involved. Ease yourself to sleep in the knowledge that you have opened the space for peace in your life today. Be grateful.

Sweet dreams...

19th day-

This morning allow your 10 breaths to just happen with your eyes closed. As you're breathing, observe how your body is naturally breathing without any guidance whatsoever. Feel the freedom in letting the breaths flow in their natural state. Be aware of how much your breath has become a source of ease in the past couple of weeks. Be grateful.

You have become familiar with "compare", "complain" and "control". The last of the 4 "c's" is "criticize". Today be aware of any criticism which comes up in your mind. Be aware of any need to criticize yourself or others. When this happens, shift your thoughts. Deliberately turn away from that and turn your thoughts toward finding the good instead of the bad. Build up, don't tear down. You have a choice. Exercise that choice in coming from a place of love instead of fear of lacking. You and everyone around you are doing the best you can. Be kind. Above all be grateful.

Enjoy your day.

Tonight, before you begin your 10 breaths, take a moment to recall an instance in which you refrained from criticizing and shifted your thoughts and attitude. How did it feel? The love that comes with allowing yourself and others to be just the way they/you are, will shift your perspective to the importance of being genuine. Ease yourself to sleep in the knowledge that you have opened the space for love in your life today. Be grateful.

Sweet dreams...

20th day-

I have to take a moment to talk about what you've been doing for the past 4 days. You have uncovered the "4 C's" - compare, complain, control and criticize. I hope you take seriously the negative impact they have in your life. Being mindful of them in your day to day dealings will have a beautiful effect on your life. Let go of them as much as you can. Some days will be easier than others. That's ok. The first step is being aware of them and the impact they have on your life. Allow yourself to come from your heart and not from a place of fear of lacking. Being everyone's best friend is not the point. Knowing that we are all different and respecting these differences is the key. On the other hand, being your own best friend is the point and even more key. Follow your intuition and do what makes you whole and gives you peace.

This morning allow your 10 breaths to just happen with your eyes closed. As you're breathing, observe how your body is naturally breathing. Feel the freedom of allowing the breath to flow effortlessly. Be aware of how much your breath has become a source of ease in the past few of weeks. Be grateful.

Today, be aware of your connection with everyone you meet, strangers or friends. Before you say anything to them, mentally say "the light which shines in me is the same light which shines in you." Be genuine in thought. It might be the checker at the grocery store, or one of your family members. Be aware of that connection. Know that you are connected to every being on this planet. Know that the same love that is you is also them.

Enjoy your day...

Tonight, I think you will find your day in review will be quite remarkable. Go over your day and how people reacted to you today after

or during your mental message to them. How did you feel? The difference your intention made in others today made life around you much better for everyone. Let your ten breaths flow effortlessly. Ease yourself to sleep in the knowledge that you have opened the space for ease in your life today. Be grateful.

Sweet dreams...

Namaste-the light which shines in me is also the light which shines in you.

21st day-

Think of three people who have had a big influence in your life, and to whom you are very grateful. Think of the ways in which they influenced you. As you take your ten breaths let gratitude settle in your every breath. Take your breaths effortlessly.

Enjoy your day...

Go a step further and write a gratitude letter to one of those people. Tell them how they have influenced you and how that has affected your life. Speak from your heart. This is especially powerful if it is written to someone whom you don't think you have thanked properly. Then either mail the letter to them, or even better, call them and read it to them. Let the love for them be expressed in gratitude.

Before you begin your ten breaths tonight, let the love and gratitude expressed in that letter fill you heart. Feel the power of love and gratitude as they go hand in hand. There is nothing that can match it. Ease yourself to sleep in the knowledge that you have opened the space for love in your life today. Be grateful.

Sweet dreams...

Namaste-the love which is in me, is the love which is in you.

22nd day-

Continue with your 10 breaths this morning. Before you start them, know that all who you met yesterday were doing the best they could, in the best way they knew how. Including you. As you breathe, give thanks for who you are and where you are. You are blessed.

Enjoy your day...

Is there someone that you haven't talked to because you had a falling out? Would you like to talk to them? If so, it's time to mend fences. Call them and extend your hand in friendship. Remember that holding on to grudges only hurts the person holding them. Try to mend a friendship fence today, and feel the lightness set in for you and them. Come from a place of love and not of fear.

If you were able to mend a fence of friendship let that feeling of love settle in to every cell of your body as you take your ten breaths tonight. If your weren't able to, mentally speak the words you would have said, if you had the chance. Ease yourself to sleep in the knowledge that you have opened a space of love for someone else. In doing so you have opened a place of serenity for yourself.

Sweet dreams...

Namaste -the light which shines in me is also the light that shines in you.

23rd day-

A moment of self-compassion can change your entire day. A string of such moments can change the course of your life.-Christopher K. Germer

We had the 4 C's to release. Now it's time for the most important "C"-Compassion. Compassion is key to leading a complete life. It needs to start with compassion for yourself. In releasing all the negative chatter for ourselves, we open the door to a place of compassion, love and kindness. We open ourselves to rest in our hearts. Then the doors and windows of our hearts can open to compassion and love for those around us. We are complete...

As you begin your ten breaths today, think of 3 ways in which you will be compassionate with yourself. As you perform your breaths allow your intention to settle into the breaths and every cell of your body.

Enjoy your day...

Be aware of your intention to be compassionate with yourself and be mindful of doing so today.

Tonight, go over your day in your mind. Go over how it felt to be compassionate with yourself. Let that feeling settle in your heart. As you take your breaths, breathe in with gratitude and as you breathe out, breathe out with love. Let only those thoughts be with you as you take your breaths. Ease yourself to sleep in the knowledge that you have opened a space to take care, nourish and love yourself unconditionally; with compassion.

Sweet dreams...

Namaste-the place for compassion in me, is also the place for compassion in you.

24th day-

Today take your ten breaths in as peaceful and serene environment as you can. Then close your eyes and do the following meditation.

First visualize yourself and say silently or out loud-

May you be healthy and strong. May you have peace in your mind, body and heart. May you be loved and love with an open heart. May you have balance, harmony and ease in everything you do. May your light shine brightly.

Secondly, visualize a loved one and repeat those words or similar sentiments in your own words.

Thirdly visualize someone you don't know very well and do the same.

After that visualize someone you don't like and wish them well in the same way.

Lastly, visualize our planet and all of these people and the rest of the beings all over the world and either repeat the words or wish for us what you would like to see.

Fully invest yourself in this meditation. Then, sit quietly for a few minutes before you get up.

Enjoy your day.

Tonight follow the same procedure you did this morning; beginning with the breaths and followed by the meditation. Ease yourself to sleep in the knowledge you have opened your heart fully to this amazing life of ours.

Sweet dreams...

Namaste-that place of unconditional love in me, is the same place of unconditional love in you.

25th day-

As you sit to practice your 10 breaths this morning, be aware of how blessed you are. think of three reasons you are blessed. With every breath let the miracle of those blessings be with you.

Enjoy your day...

It's a day of counting blessings. Do not let an opportunity get by you, no matter how small it is, to see the blessing it is. Where the focus goes, is where the energy goes. Focus on those little miracles around you and you will create more miracles. Your breath alone is a form of miracle, if you take the time to really see how incredible the process is.

Before taking your ten breaths tonight, think of three different miracles which you were blessed with today. Let the beauty of them settle into every breath. Ease yourself to sleep in the knowledge that you are blessed and have made the space for more blessings.

Sweet dreams...

Namaste-the miracle I am, is also the miracle you are.

26th day-

As you sit today for your ten breaths, be aware of receiving the breaths as you're inhaling and also be aware of sharing the breaths as you're exhaling. Practice receiving and giving your breaths with a full heart.

Enjoy your day...

The cycle of breathing is one of giving and receiving of much importance to us, but also to our planet as a whole. Your breath makes a difference to you as you receive and nourish. Without it you couldn't survive. But think of the importance of your exhalation. Without it the plant life around you would not survive. Our interdependence is a vital process of survival through receiving and giving. We have all studied this in school somewhere along the way, but have we realized our true importance in simply breathing? Take moments throughout your day today to be with your breath, knowing the difference the cycle makes; a cycle that would not be possible without you. Go outside and kick off your shoes in the grass, dirt or sand and ground yourself with the earth below you. Feel how much a part of it you are. Be aware of the miracles of life and your part in that.

Tonight, go over how your feet felt touching the ground below you, with the knowledge of the connection and the importance of you in this world. While practicing your ten breaths, do so with full awareness of the importance of receiving. In life, without receiving, giving would not be possible; not just in breathing. Unless we are open to receiving we have nothing to give. Invite and accept blessings to fill your being. Ease yourself to sleep in the knowledge that you are important to this world and have made the space for receiving.

Sweet dreams...

Namaste- the importance of my being, is the same importance of your being.

27th day-

As you get ready to take your 10 breaths this morning, sit silently and bring your awareness to your thoughts. Don't try to change them, just be aware of them, and observe them as they come and as they go. Observe your mind with the mind in your heart, without judgement, simply watch the thoughts come and go. As you start your breaths, visualize and try to feel the breaths coming in through your heart and as you exhale feel the breaths leaving through your heart. Let the focus go from the thoughts to the breath. Be grateful.

Enjoy your day...

Take time to be with your thoughts throughout the day. Simply observe them in the way you did this morning. As you observe them, try not to judge them, just watch them as they come and go. Notice how once you drop judgement, and observe as if you are a third person, your thoughts no longer have an effect on you. Take it a step further and choose to change your perspective on a thought which might be causing you distress. Shifting perspective without judgement will free you of any expectation or worries and allow you to accept what is, in a way you may not have before. The moment you release your emotional expectations, you release yourself and others and the energy becomes simple and free.

Be kind to yourself tonight. As you sit down for your ten breaths, think of all the thoughts you observed today. Label them. Know that no matter what the label is, it's ok. Love yourself unconditionally through those thoughts, and in that way you can experience that unconditional love with others. It all begins from within.

In gratitude and compassion for the being that you are, begin your ten breaths and visualize the inhalation through your heart and as you exhale feel the breath leaving through your heart. Ease yourself to sleep in the knowledge that your thoughts are not who you are, and that you have made the space for compassion and love. Be grateful.

Sweet dreams...

Namaste- the love in me is beyond thoughts, in the same way the love in you is.

28th day-

As I'm writing this today I am thinking of all the processes we have been through. Each day, I have tried to give you a different perspective in a different way. The one constant that hasn't varied has been taking time for your daily breaths. I can't stress enough the importance of the breath. It will take you within and will guide you to find your own answers as you need them.

Today sit with your back straight, your neck straight and your eyes gently closed. Place your palms in your lap with the right palm supporting the left palm and the thumbs gently touching each other. As you breathe in, breathe in through your nose and as you breathe out, breathe out through your lips. Don't try to control the breath, just let it flow with ease. Now, I want you to visualize and not just in your mind's eye, but "feel" the breath coming in though your heart as you're breathing in and as you're breathing out, feel it leaving through your heart. Continue to breathe through your heart and feel the continuous flow of energy passing through your heart. As you breathe in, breathe in with love and as you breathe out share that love. As you breathe in, think of someone you love and as you breathe out feel yourself sharing your love with them with the breath out. As you continue to breathe, feel free to bring other people whom you love to mind and do the same with them in mind. If you feel

like having more than 10 breaths today, by all means do so. As you finish your breaths, visualize giving those breaths to yourself in love and with compassion. Feel the peace and balance that comes with allowing yourself to feel that love. Sit silently with your eyes closed once you're finished and allow the process to settle in every cell of your body and mind. There is no goal here. Just be.

Enjoy your day...

Some time during the day today, breathe through your heart. You don't have to close your eyes, if it's not possible to do so.

Tonight, be aware of how breathing through your heart has made you feel for the past two days. In gratitude and with full intention practice your ten breaths in the same way you did this morning. Ease yourself to sleep in the knowledge that you love and you are loved.

Sweet dreams...

Namaste- the love that lies in my heart, is the same love which lies in yours.

29th day-

You have been breathing through your heart and I hope you were able to feel the infinite love within you. Continue to do so and you will feel the expansion happen without any effort. Let's take your breath work a little further today.

Sit with your back straight, your neck straight and your eyes gently closed. Place your palms in your lap with the right palm supporting the left palm and the thumbs gently touching each other. As you breathe in, breathe in through your nose and as you breathe out, breathe out through your lips. Don't try to control the breath, just let it flow with ease. Now, I want you to visualize and not just in your mind's eye, but "feel" the breath coming in though your heart as you're breathing in and as you're breathing out, feel it leaving through your heart. Continue to breathe through your heart and feel the continuous flow of energy passing through your heart. As you breathe in, breathe in with gratitude and as you breathe out, do so with gratitude. As you breathe in, think of someone you are grateful for and as you breathe out feel yourself sharing your gratitude with them with the breath out. As you continue to breathe, feel free to bring other people for whom you are grateful to mind and do the same with them in mind. If you feel like having more than 10 breaths today, please do so. As you finish, visualize those breaths for you and the beautiful being you are, with gratitude and with compassion. Feel the joy and ease that comes with allowing yourself to be grateful. Sit silently with your eyes closed once you're finished and allow the process to settle in every cell of your body and mind. There is no goal here. Just be.

Bring gratitude to it's rightful place in your heart and stand back and watch magic happen.

Enjoy your day…

Today find at least three moments in which to be grateful. If you think you have nothing to be grateful for, continue your search throughout your day until you find that moment. Don't stop there. Continue your search. It's not gratitude that matters most; it's the searching for it that makes the difference. It's a real shift in perspective when your heart and mind come together to go through the day searching and finding that for which to be grateful. Before you know it, it becomes your nature. Where the focus goes is where the energy goes. If the focus is on gratitude then that is where your mind and heart will go. Guide them.

Tonight I hope your heart will be so full that you will be taking your ten breaths with a sense of wholeness. Allow them to happen spontaneously and watch the difference that focus made on your life today. Breathing in gratitude means you are living in gratitude. Ease yourself to sleep in the knowledge that you have uncovered that place within your heart and mind where gratitude thrives.

Sweet dreams...

Namaste- the place of gratitude within me, is the same place of gratitude within you.

30th day-

We touched a little on being in the moment, and I can't let you go without guiding you through the process of living the moment. Our life is made of moments, literally. As you finished reading this sentence a moment has passed. How we choose to spend our moments, and more importantly, how we choose to be part of our moments makes all the difference in the meaning of our lives. Think about your thoughts in any given day. A large part of them are thoughts of what will happen or what did happen. Seldom are they completely related to what you are doing at any given moment with complete awareness.

At this moment in time you are safe and fed and probably sitting comfortably. Be grateful.

Before you begin your breaths today, I would like you to sit with your back straight, neck straight and hands in your lap with the right palm supporting the left palm and the thumbs gently touching each other. Take a few breaths with your own natural rhythm. Begin to focus on the ground below you, the space around you and where you are in relation to everything around you. Even though your eyes are closed, scan the room you are in and know where everything is. Be aware of how safe you are. Be aware that at this moment in time you have nothing to worry about. At this moment in time it is just you and your breath. Begin your ten breath process and as you breathe in, breathe in through your nose and breathe out through your lips. Then shift your focus to your heart and feel the breath flowing through your heart. As you are doing this, be aware of this moment in time. Be aware of the gift of this moment in time. Be aware that each breath is a moment of time which is precious and important in it's own right. Only be aware of "now". Only be aware of being alive and breathing and safe "now", in this moment in time. When you have finished your breaths, allow some time to sit in silence. Be grateful

Enjoy your day...

Today, when you wash your hands focus on the moments you are spending washing your hands. Focus on how the soap feels on your skin; what the water temperature is and how it feels as it washes the soap off your skin. As you dry your hands be aware of how the towel feels and how your muscles feel holding the towel. Focus on every part of washing your hands. Be conscious of the present moment in washing your hands and all the movements and muscles it takes to do so. If you can do it with your eyes closed it will add extra depth to your experience. Do this every time you wash your hands today.

Tonight sit in the same way you did this morning. Bring your attention to "now", to the present moment and practice your ten breaths with full awareness of how your body feels with every breath. Experience how your heart feels as the energy flows through it and how your mind feels experiencing all your senses. Be grateful

You have spent moments today being completely present in the "now". "Now" is all we have. Don't let it get away from you in the "what was" or "what might be." What's done is done and the past is gone. The future is yours to have and there is no use worrying about things which will most likely never happen. Focus on what you have "now", not what you don't have. Know that you are exactly where you need to be at this and at any given moment in time. Ease yourself to sleep in the knowledge that the present moment is yours and you are rich because of it. Be grateful for this moment in time.

Sweet dreams...

Namaste- the beauty of my moments is the same beauty your moments hold.

31st day-

Today is our last day. For those of you who were with me every day, I hope I did you justice. For those who popped in and out, I know that you popped in exactly when you needed it and I hope you received what you needed. I thank you all for being part of this journey.

Our lives are made up of moments. In order to truly live and appreciate this life, we need to be in those moments. Release the past without guilt, plan for the future with joy, and live the present moment with genuine presence and gratitude. Accept and let go of expecting. Release the 4 "C's"-comparison, complaint, control, and criticism, and instead embrace the big "C"-Compassion. Do this for yourself and all those around you. Be grateful for you and who you are and live through that gratitude in a genuine state as you take "should" out of your vocabulary. And most of all, no matter what you do, do it from your heart.

Today, let's sit together as we have done once before.

Take your ten breaths in as peaceful and serene environment as you can. Then close your eyes and do the following meditation.

First visualize yourself and say silently or out loud-

May you be healthy and strong. May you have peace in your mind, body and heart. May you be loved and love with an open heart. May you have balance, harmony and ease in everything you do. May your light shine brightly.

Secondly, visualize a loved one and repeat those words or similar sentiments in your own words.

Thirdly visualize someone you don't know very well and do the same.

After that visualize someone you don't like and wish them well in the same way.

Lastly, visualize our planet and all of these people and the rest of the beings all over the world and either repeat the words or wish for us what you would like to see.

Fully invest yourself in this meditation. Then, sit quietly for a few minutes before you get up.

Enjoy your day...

Today reflect but don't regret. Every decision you have made has brought you to this moment in time. What we perceive as mistakes are lessons. Review your life in gratitude and move through today with awareness.

Tonight, take 1 breath in gratitude as you're easing yourself to sleep in the knowledge that you are finishing this journey to peace with awareness of this moment and breath and all moments to come.

Sweet dreams...

Namaste- the light of love which shines brightly in me, is the same loving bright light which shines in you.

Made in the USA
Middletown, DE
09 March 2021